I0458644

Kidney Patient's Complete Low Potassium Cookbook

Flavorful Recipes for Kidney Health Manage Your Diet with Delicious, Low-Potassium Meals and Tips

Janeth Kingston BSN RN

DISCLAIMER

The information, including but not limited to, text, graphics, images and other material contained in this guide are for informational purposes only. No material from this guide is intended to be a substitute for professional medical advice, diagnosis or treatment.

Always seek the advice of your physician or other qualified health care provider with any questions you may have regarding a medical condition or treatment and before undertaking a new health care regimen, and never disregard professional medical advice or delay in seeking it because of something you have read in this guide.

Table of CONTENTS

INTRODUCTION

Welcome to the Essential Low Potassium Cookbook

Welcome to The Essential Low Potassium Cookbook: Flavorful Recipes for Kidney Health! This book is your comprehensive guide to navigating the complexities of a low-potassium diet while still enjoying delicious and satisfying meals. Whether you are managing chronic kidney disease (CKD), heart disease, or dietary restrictions, this cookbook is designed to empower you with the knowledge and tools you need to thrive.

Why This Cookbook?
Living with dietary restrictions can often feel overwhelming. Many individuals and families struggle to find meals that are both nutritious and flavorful while adhering to specific dietary guidelines. With this cookbook, we aim to change that narrative. Our goal is to provide you with a variety of recipes that not only meet low-potassium requirements but also excite your palate. In this cookbook, you will discover:

- **Understanding Potassium and Kidney Health:** A thorough explanation of what potassium is, its significance in kidney function, and the conditions that require potassium management.

- **The Basics of a Low Potassium Diet:** Key principles, cooking techniques, and tips to help you successfully implement a low-potassium diet into your daily routine.

- **Delicious Recipes:** An array of flavorful recipes for breakfast, lunch, dinner, and snacks, all carefully crafted to be low in potassium without sacrificing taste. From hearty soups to delightful desserts, there's something for everyone!

- **Meal Planning for Success:** Practical advice on creating meal plans and prepping low-potassium meals to make it easier to stay on track with your dietary goals.

- **Coping with Dietary Restrictions:** Strategies for navigating social situations, cooking for families with mixed dietary needs, and involving loved ones in meal preparation.

A Message from Janeth Kingston

As a nephrology nurse with over a decade of experience, I understand the challenges that come with managing dietary restrictions. My mission is to help you take control of your health while enjoying the foods you love. With the right knowledge and support, you can navigate your CKD journey confidently and live a full, vibrant life.

Thank you for choosing The Essential Low Potassium Cookbook. Let's embark on this culinary journey together, transforming the way you think about food and health. Here's to delicious meals that promote your well-being!

Bon Appétit!

Janeth Kingston's Story

My journey into the world of nephrology and dietary management began over a decade ago when I first started my career as a registered nurse. With a Bachelor of Science in Nursing (BSN) and a passion for helping others, I quickly found my niche in the field of nephrology. My work has taken me across the United States and Europe, where I have had the privilege of supporting countless patients dealing with chronic kidney disease (CKD) and related health challenges.

Discovering My Passion

Early in my nursing career, I noticed a significant gap in resources available for patients managing their diets, particularly when it came to understanding potassium levels. Many of my patients expressed frustration about feeling restricted in their food choices and were overwhelmed by the complexities of a low-potassium diet. This realization sparked a passion in me to empower patients with knowledge and practical tools to improve their quality of life.

Commitment to Education

Recognizing the importance of education in patient care, I began collaborating with nephrology researchers, kidney-specialized chefs, and leading nephrologists to develop comprehensive dietary resources.

Throughout my career, I have been dedicated to patient education and support. Since 2017, I have guided CKD patients, helping them navigate dietary management, understand the significance of potassium control, and regain confidence in their food choices. I've seen firsthand how the right knowledge can empower individuals to take control of their health.

The Birth of This Cookbook

The idea for The Essential Low Potassium Cookbook was born from my desire to provide a comprehensive guide that combines my nursing experience with my passion for cooking. I wanted to create a resource that offers not just recipes, but also a deeper understanding of the relationship between diet and kidney health.

This cookbook is a culmination of years of experience, research, and feedback from patients. It is designed to be practical and approachable, ensuring that anyone can create delicious, low-potassium meals without sacrificing flavor or enjoyment.

Looking Ahead

As I continue my journey in nephrology, my mission remains clear: to empower individuals with the knowledge and resources they need to navigate their dietary needs confidently. I believe that with the right support, anyone can lead a fulfilling and vibrant life, even while managing chronic health conditions.

Thank you for joining me on this journey. I hope that The Essential Low Potassium Cookbook becomes a valuable resource in your kitchen, inspiring you to explore the world of low-potassium cooking with joy and creativity. Together, we can transform the way we think about food and health!

HOW TO BEST USE THIS 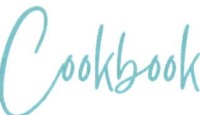 Cookbook

Welcome to The Essential Low Potassium Cookbook! This book is designed to be a valuable resource for anyone looking to navigate a low-potassium diet while still enjoying delicious and satisfying meals. Here are some tips and guidelines to help you make the most of this cookbook:

- **Understand Your Dietary Needs:** Before diving into the recipes, take the time to familiarize yourself with your specific dietary requirements. Consult with your healthcare provider or a registered dietitian to understand your potassium limits and any other dietary restrictions you may have.
- **Explore the Introduction:** Start with the introductory sections, including Understanding Potassium and Kidney Health and The Basics of a Low Potassium Diet. These sections provide essential information about potassium, its impact on kidney health, and foundational principles for managing a low-potassium diet.
- **Use the Table of Contents:** The Table of Contents is organized by meal types (breakfast, lunch, dinner, snacks, and desserts) and topics such as meal planning and coping with dietary restrictions. Use it to quickly find recipes that suit your needs and mealtime preferences.
- **Browse Recipes:** Feel free to browse through the recipes to discover new dishes you might enjoy. Each recipe includes nutritional information, preparation time, and serving suggestions, making it easy to plan your meals.
- **Plan Your Meals:** Take advantage of the meal planning tips provided in the Meal Planning for Success section. Consider creating a weekly meal plan that incorporates a variety of recipes from different categories. This will help you stay organized and ensure you're meeting your dietary goals.

- **Customize Recipes:** Many recipes can be customized to suit your taste preferences and dietary needs. Feel free to adjust ingredient quantities, swap out vegetables, or substitute proteins as long as they fit within your potassium limits. This flexibility allows you to make the recipes your own.
- **Involve Family and Friends:** Cooking can be a fun and engaging activity. Involve family members or friends in the meal preparation process. This not only makes cooking more enjoyable but also helps educate others about your dietary needs and preferences.
- **Experiment with New Ingredients:** Use this cookbook as an opportunity to explore new ingredients and cooking techniques. Discovering low-potassium alternatives or trying out new spices can enhance the flavor of your meals and keep your diet interesting.
- **Stay Organized:** Keep a list of your favorite recipes and any adjustments you make to them. This will help you streamline your cooking process and ensure you always have go-to meals that satisfy your taste buds and dietary needs.
- **Seek Support:** If you find navigating a low-potassium diet challenging, don't hesitate to reach out for support. Join online communities, support groups, or educational workshops focused on kidney health and dietary management. Sharing experiences and tips with others can be incredibly helpful.

Remember, this cookbook is here to support you on your journey to better health. While managing a low-potassium diet may feel overwhelming at times, with the right resources and knowledge, you can enjoy flavorful meals that nourish your body. Embrace the process, try new things, and most importantly, enjoy the journey of cooking and eating well!

Happy Cooking!

Why Janeth Kingston is an Authority on Kidney Health and Nutrition

Janeth Kingston, BSN, RN, is a recognized expert in the field of nephrology and dietary management for individuals with chronic kidney disease (CKD). Her extensive background, professional experiences, and commitment to patient education make her a trusted authority in kidney health and nutrition. Here are several key reasons why Janeth is highly regarded in this field:

Extensive Clinical Experience
With over a decade of experience as a nephrology nurse, Janeth has worked directly with thousands of patients diagnosed with kidney disease. Her hands-on experience in clinical settings has provided her with valuable insights into the challenges and needs of individuals managing CKD and related health conditions.

Focus on Dietary Management
Janeth has dedicated her career to understanding the intricate relationship between diet and kidney health. She has collaborated with nephrologists, researchers, and dietitians to develop evidence-based dietary guidelines tailored for patients requiring potassium management. Her expertise in dietary restrictions empowers her to create practical and delicious recipes that meet the nutritional needs of those with CKD.

Patient-Centric Approach
Janeth's empathetic approach to patient care sets her apart as a healthcare provider. She understands the emotional and psychological challenges faced by patients dealing with dietary restrictions, and she prioritizes education and support. By empowering her patients with knowledge about their health and dietary choices, she helps them regain control over their lives.

Commitment to Lifelong Learning
Janeth's dedication to continuous education and professional development ensures that she stays updated on the latest advancements in kidney health and nutrition. Her commitment to lifelong learning translates into improved care for her patients and a deeper understanding of nutritional strategies that can enhance their quality of life.

Janeth Kingston's extensive clinical experience, focus on dietary management, recognized research contributions, patient-centric approach, and commitment to education make her an authority on kidney health and nutrition. Through her work, she empowers individuals with CKD to make informed dietary choices that support their health and well-being. Her passion for improving the lives of those living with kidney disease is evident in every aspect of her career, making her a trusted ally in the CKD community.

Background in Nursing and Nephrology

Janeth Kingston's journey in nursing and nephrology is a testament to her dedication, expertise, and passion for improving the lives of individuals living with chronic kidney disease (CKD). Her background encompasses a wealth of clinical experience, education, and a commitment to patient advocacy that positions her as a leading authority in the field. Here are the key elements of her background in nursing and nephrology:

Educational Foundation
Janeth earned her Bachelor of Science in Nursing (BSN) from a reputable nursing program, equipping her with the foundational knowledge and skills necessary for a successful nursing career. This education paved the way for her specialization in nephrology, where she would go on to make a significant impact.

Clinical Experience
With over a decade of experience as a registered nurse, Janeth has worked in various clinical settings, including hospitals, outpatient clinics, and dialysis centers. Her hands-on experience with patients suffering from kidney disease has provided her with valuable insights into the complexities of managing CKD and its associated complications.

Specialization in Nephrology
Janeth's focus on nephrology began early in her career, fueled by her desire to understand the unique challenges faced by patients with kidney disease. She has developed expertise in various aspects of nephrology, including the physiological and nutritional needs of her patients. This specialization has allowed her to become a trusted resource for patients and healthcare professionals alike.

Patient Education and Support
A significant part of Janeth's role as a nephrology nurse has involved patient education. She understands that many patients feel overwhelmed by their diagnosis and the dietary restrictions that come with managing kidney health. Janeth is dedicated to empowering her patients by providing clear, accessible information about their conditions and the importance of dietary management, fostering a supportive environment where patients feel heard and understood.

Continued Professional Development
Janeth is dedicated to lifelong learning and professional development. She regularly participates in continuing education opportunities, workshops, and conferences to stay current with the latest advancements in nephrology and nursing practice. This commitment to ongoing education enhances her ability to provide the best possible care to her patients.

Janeth Kingston's background in nursing and nephrology is characterized by her extensive clinical experience, dedication to patient education, and commitment to improving the lives of individuals with chronic kidney disease. Her holistic approach to care, combined with her advocacy efforts and collaborative spirit, positions her as a leader in the field. Through her work, Janeth continues to inspire and empower patients to take control of their health and navigate their CKD journey with confidence.

Experience in Dietary Management for Potassium Control

Janeth Kingston's extensive experience in dietary management for potassium control is a cornerstone of her expertise in nephrology and patient care. Her commitment to empowering individuals with chronic kidney disease (CKD) through effective dietary strategies has been shaped by years of clinical practice, collaboration with healthcare professionals, and a deep understanding of the complexities of potassium management. Here are the key aspects of her experience in this vital area:

Patient-Centered Dietary Education
Janeth has dedicated a significant portion of her nursing career to educating patients about the importance of potassium management. She recognizes that many individuals with CKD feel overwhelmed by their dietary restrictions and the need to monitor potassium intake. Through one-on-one consultations and group education sessions, Janeth provides clear, accessible information about potassium, its role in kidney health, and how to effectively manage dietary choices.

Customized Meal Planning
Understanding that each patient has unique dietary needs, Janeth works closely with individuals to develop customized meal plans that align with their potassium restrictions while still being enjoyable and satisfying. She emphasizes the importance of incorporating a variety of foods that are low in potassium and rich in flavor, ensuring that patients do not feel deprived of delicious meals.

Recipe Development and Resources
Recognizing the challenges of finding tasty, low-potassium recipes, Janeth has been actively involved in developing and curating a collection of recipes that meet potassium management guidelines. Her cookbook, The Essential Low Potassium Cookbook, includes a variety of flavorful recipes that empower patients to cook with confidence while adhering to their dietary restrictions.

Research and Evidence-Based Practices
Janeth stays informed about the latest research and evidence-based practices related to dietary management for potassium control. She actively incorporates new findings into her patient education and meal planning strategies, ensuring that her patients benefit from the most current and effective dietary approaches.

Long-Term Follow-up and Support
Janeth believes in the importance of long-term follow-up and support for individuals managing CKD. She regularly checks in with her patients to assess their dietary adherence, address challenges, and make necessary adjustments to their meal plans. This ongoing support is crucial for maintaining dietary compliance and improving overall health outcomes.

Janeth Kingston's experience in dietary management for potassium control is characterized by her patient-centered approach, collaboration with healthcare professionals, and commitment to empowering individuals with chronic kidney disease. Through education, customized meal planning, and ongoing support, Janeth helps her patients navigate the complexities of a low-potassium diet, ensuring they can enjoy flavorful meals while successfully managing their health. Her expertise not only enhances the lives of her patients but also contributes to a broader understanding of the critical role nutrition plays in kidney health.

Commitment to Patient Education and Support

Janeth Kingston's commitment to patient education and support is a defining aspect of her career as a nephrology nurse and a trusted advocate for individuals managing chronic kidney disease (CKD). Understanding that knowledge is power, Janeth has dedicated herself to empowering patients with the information and resources they need to take control of their health. Here are key elements of her commitment to patient education and support:

Empowering Through Knowledge
Janeth believes that educating patients about their condition is crucial for effective self-management. She provides clear, evidence-based information about CKD, its progression, and the importance of diet in managing potassium levels.

Development of Educational Materials
Janeth has created a variety of educational materials, including brochures, handouts, and online resources, that simplify complex information about CKD and dietary management. These materials serve as valuable tools for patients and their families, making it easier to understand dietary guidelines and potassium management.

Support for Caregivers and Families
Understanding that the journey of managing CKD can be challenging not only for patients but also for their caregivers, Janeth extends her educational efforts to families and support networks. She provides guidance on how caregivers can best support their loved ones, emphasizing the importance of a collaborative approach to health management.

Utilizing Technology

Embracing modern technology, Janeth utilizes digital platforms to reach a broader audience. She shares valuable insights, recipes, and tips through social media and online forums, making kidney health education accessible to individuals who may not have the opportunity to attend in-person sessions.

Janeth Kingston's unwavering commitment to patient education and support is a cornerstone of her approach to nephrology nursing. By empowering individuals with knowledge, providing personalized education, and fostering a supportive community, she helps patients navigate the complexities of chronic kidney disease with confidence. Her dedication not only enhances the lives of her patients but also contributes to a culture of understanding and compassion within the healthcare system, ensuring that those living with CKD have the resources they need to thrive.

Understanding

POTASSIUM AND KIDNEY HEALTH

What is Potassium and Why is it Important?

What is Potassium and Why is it Important?
Potassium is an essential mineral and electrolyte that plays a crucial role in various bodily functions. It is vital for maintaining overall health and well-being, especially for individuals with certain health conditions, such as chronic kidney disease (CKD). Understanding potassium's functions and its importance can help individuals manage their diets effectively.

What is Potassium?
Potassium is a naturally occurring mineral found in many foods and is essential for multiple physiological processes in the body. It is one of the key electrolytes, along with sodium, calcium, and magnesium, that help regulate fluid balance, muscle contractions, and nerve signals.

Sources of Potassium
Potassium is abundant in many foods, including:
- Fruits: Bananas, oranges, apricots, and avocados
- Vegetables: Spinach, potatoes, sweet potatoes, and tomatoes
- Legumes: Beans and lentils
- Dairy Products: Milk and yogurt
- Nuts and Seeds: Almonds, peanuts, and sunflower seeds

Why is Potassium Important?
- Regulation of Fluid Balance
  - Potassium helps maintain the balance of fluids in and out of cells, tissues, and organs. This balance is essential for proper hydration and overall bodily function.
- Muscle Function
  - Potassium plays a vital role in muscle contraction. It helps transmit electrical signals that facilitate muscle movement, including the heart muscle. Adequate potassium levels are crucial for normal muscle function and preventing cramps.

- Nerve Impulse Transmission
  - Potassium is essential for proper nerve function. It helps transmit electrical impulses between nerve cells, enabling communication throughout the nervous system. This function is critical for reflexes, coordination, and overall nervous system health.
- Heart Health
  - Potassium is important for maintaining a healthy heart rhythm. It helps regulate blood pressure by counteracting the effects of sodium, promoting vasodilation, and reducing strain on the cardiovascular system. Adequate potassium intake is associated with a lower risk of hypertension and cardiovascular disease.
- Acid-Base Balance
  - Potassium helps maintain the body's acid-base balance, which is vital for normal cellular function. It assists in regulating pH levels in the blood, which is essential for optimal metabolic processes.

Potassium and Chronic Kidney Disease (CKD)

For individuals with CKD, managing potassium intake becomes especially important. The kidneys play a crucial role in regulating potassium levels in the body. When kidney function declines, the ability to excrete excess potassium diminishes, which can lead to hyperkalemia (high potassium levels). Hyperkalemia can cause serious health issues, including heart arrhythmias and muscle weakness.

Dietary Management

For those with CKD, a low-potassium diet may be recommended to prevent the complications associated with elevated potassium levels. This involves:
- Monitoring potassium-rich foods and adjusting portion sizes.
- Incorporating low-potassium alternatives in meals.
- Understanding food preparation methods that can help reduce potassium content, such as leaching or boiling.

Potassium is a vital mineral that supports numerous bodily functions, from fluid regulation to muscle contraction and nerve transmission. While it is essential for health, individuals with chronic kidney disease must carefully manage their potassium intake to prevent complications. Understanding the role of potassium and its importance can empower individuals to make informed dietary choices that promote their health and well-being.

The Role of Potassium
in Kidney Function

Potassium is an essential mineral that plays a significant role in maintaining various physiological functions in the body, particularly in relation to kidney health. The kidneys are responsible for regulating potassium levels in the body, and understanding this relationship is crucial for individuals with chronic kidney disease (CKD) or other related conditions. Here's a closer look at the role of potassium in kidney function:

1. Regulation of Electrolyte Balance

- *Electrolyte Homeostasis:* Potassium is one of the key electrolytes in the body, along with sodium, calcium, and magnesium. It is vital for maintaining the balance of fluids and electrolytes in and out of cells, tissues, and organs. The kidneys help regulate this balance by adjusting the amount of potassium excreted in urine.
- *Sodium-Potassium Relationship:* Potassium works in tandem with sodium to maintain fluid balance and blood pressure. When sodium levels increase, potassium levels can help counteract the effects by promoting sodium excretion through urine.

2. Muscle and Nerve Function

- *Muscle Contraction:* Potassium is essential for muscle function, including the contraction of the heart muscle. The kidneys help maintain appropriate potassium levels, which are critical for normal muscle contractions and overall cardiovascular health.
- *Nerve Impulse Transmission:* Potassium plays a crucial role in the transmission of nerve impulses. It helps generate and conduct electrical signals between nerve cells, enabling communication throughout the nervous system. Proper kidney function is necessary to maintain these potassium levels, ensuring optimal nerve function.

3. Acid-Base Balance

- *pH Regulation:* Potassium is involved in maintaining the body's acid-base balance (pH level). The kidneys contribute to this balance by regulating the excretion of hydrogen ions and bicarbonate in relation to potassium levels. This regulation is vital for normal metabolic processes and overall health.

4. Impact of Kidney Dysfunction on Potassium Regulation

- *Impaired Excretion:* In individuals with CKD, the kidneys' ability to filter and excrete potassium diminishes. This can lead to an accumulation of potassium in the bloodstream, a condition known as hyperkalemia. Elevated potassium levels can have serious consequences, including muscle weakness, fatigue, and potentially life-threatening heart arrhythmias.
- *Dietary Management:* For individuals with CKD, managing dietary potassium intake becomes essential to prevent hyperkalemia. This often involves restricting high-potassium foods and following a low-potassium diet, as well as regular monitoring of potassium levels through blood tests.

5. Potassium as a Nutrient for Kidney Health

- *Balanced Intake:* While potassium restriction is crucial for individuals with kidney dysfunction, it's important to note that potassium is still an essential nutrient for overall health. For those with healthy kidneys, adequate potassium intake is necessary for maintaining normal bodily functions, including muscle contractions, nerve function, and blood pressure regulation.
- *Low-Potassium Alternatives:* For individuals who need to reduce their potassium intake, there are many low-potassium food alternatives available that can help maintain a balanced diet without compromising health.

Potassium plays a vital role in kidney function and overall health. The kidneys are responsible for regulating potassium levels in the body, and any impairment in kidney function can disrupt this balance, leading to potentially serious health issues. Understanding the relationship between potassium and kidney function is essential for individuals with CKD or other related conditions, empowering them to make informed dietary choices that promote their health and well-being. Proper management of potassium intake is crucial for preventing complications and maintaining a healthy lifestyle.

Conditions Requiring
Potassium Management

Potassium is an essential mineral that plays a critical role in various bodily functions, including muscle contractions, nerve signal transmission, and maintaining fluid balance. However, certain medical conditions can affect the body's ability to manage potassium levels effectively, leading to the need for careful dietary management. Here are some key conditions that require potassium management:

1. **Chronic Kidney Disease (CKD)**
- *Impaired Kidney Function:* In CKD, the kidneys gradually lose their ability to filter waste and excess minerals from the blood. This includes the regulation of potassium levels. As kidney function declines, potassium can accumulate in the bloodstream, leading to hyperkalemia (high potassium levels).
- *Dietary Restrictions:* Individuals with CKD often need to follow a low-potassium diet to prevent complications associated with elevated potassium levels, such as muscle weakness, fatigue, and serious heart arrhythmias.

2. **Acute Kidney Injury (AKI)**
- *Sudden Loss of Function:* AKI is characterized by a rapid decline in kidney function, which can occur due to various factors, including dehydration, infections, or certain medications. During this time, the kidneys may struggle to excrete potassium effectively.
- *Close Monitoring:* Patients with AKI may require close monitoring of potassium levels and may need dietary adjustments to manage potassium intake until kidney function improves.

3. **End-Stage Renal Disease (ESRD)**
- *Dialysis Dependence:* Individuals with ESRD have severely impaired kidney function and often require dialysis to remove waste products and excess minerals from the blood. Both hemodialysis and peritoneal dialysis can affect potassium levels, necessitating careful dietary management.
- *Potassium Restrictions:* Patients on dialysis may need to follow strict low-potassium diets to prevent hyperkalemia between treatments.

4. Heart Conditions

- *Heart Disease:* Conditions such as heart failure and arrhythmias can be affected by potassium levels. Proper potassium balance is essential for maintaining a healthy heart rhythm.
- *Medication Interactions:* Certain medications used to treat heart conditions (e.g., diuretics) can impact potassium levels, either causing depletion or contributing to retention. Patients may require potassium monitoring and dietary adjustments based on their medication regimen.

5. Medications Affecting Potassium Levels

- *Diuretics:* Some diuretics (commonly referred to as "water pills") can lead to increased potassium loss (thiazide diuretics) or potassium retention (potassium-sparing diuretics). Patients taking these medications may need to adjust their potassium intake based on their specific situation.
- *ACE Inhibitors and ARBs:* Medications used to treat high blood pressure and heart failure, such as angiotensin-converting enzyme (ACE) inhibitors and angiotensin receptor blockers (ARBs), can increase potassium levels. Patients on these medications require regular monitoring of potassium levels.

6. Hormonal Disorders

- *Adrenal Insufficiency:* Conditions like Addison's disease can result in elevated potassium levels due to insufficient production of aldosterone, a hormone that helps regulate potassium balance. Individuals with adrenal insufficiency may require potassium management to prevent complications.
- *Hyperaldosteronism:* Conversely, conditions causing excessive production of aldosterone can lead to low potassium levels (hypokalemia). Patients may need to monitor and manage their potassium intake accordingly.

7. Gastrointestinal Disorders

- *Diarrhea and Vomiting:* Conditions that cause prolonged diarrhea or vomiting can lead to significant potassium loss, resulting in hypokalemia. Individuals experiencing these conditions may require potassium supplementation or dietary adjustments to restore balance.
- *Malabsorption Disorders:* Conditions such as celiac disease or Crohn's disease can affect nutrient absorption, including potassium. Patients may need to monitor their potassium levels and dietary intake closely.

Potassium management is crucial for individuals with various medical conditions, particularly those affecting kidney function, heart health, and hormonal balance. Understanding the need for potassium regulation can help patients make informed dietary choices and prevent complications associated with elevated or depleted potassium levels. It is essential for individuals with these conditions to work closely with healthcare professionals to develop personalized dietary plans that meet their specific health needs.

The Basics of a

LOW POTASSIUM DIET

What is a Low Potassium Diet?

What is a Low Potassium Diet?

A low potassium diet is a dietary approach that restricts the intake of potassium-rich foods to help manage potassium levels in the body. This type of diet is particularly important for individuals with conditions that affect kidney function, such as chronic kidney disease (CKD), acute kidney injury (AKI), or end-stage renal disease (ESRD). By reducing potassium intake, individuals can help prevent hyperkalemia (high potassium levels), which can lead to serious health complications.

Benefits of a Low Potassium Diet

- *Prevention of Hyperkalemia:* By managing potassium intake, individuals can reduce the risk of developing hyperkalemia, which can lead to serious complications such as cardiac arrhythmias.
- *Improved Kidney Health:* For individuals with kidney disease, a low potassium diet can help support kidney function and prevent further damage.
- *Enhanced Quality of Life:* By providing tasty and satisfying meal options that comply with dietary restrictions, individuals can maintain a more enjoyable and fulfilling eating experience.

A low potassium diet is an essential dietary strategy for individuals with compromised kidney function or those at risk of hyperkalemia. By understanding which foods to limit and which to include, individuals can effectively manage their potassium levels while still enjoying a variety of flavorful meals. Collaboration with healthcare professionals is vital to ensure that dietary choices align with individual health needs and goals.

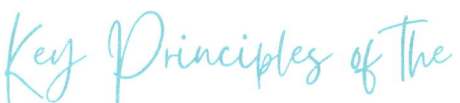
Key Principles of The

Low Potassium Diet

A low potassium diet is designed to help individuals manage their potassium intake, particularly those with chronic kidney disease (CKD), acute kidney injury (AKI), or other conditions that affect potassium regulation. Here are the key principles to consider when following a low potassium diet:

1. Understanding Potassium Sources

- *Identify High-Potassium Foods:* Familiarize yourself with foods that are high in potassium, which should be limited or avoided. Common high-potassium foods include:
  - Fruits: Bananas, oranges, apricots, avocados, and dried fruits.
  - Vegetables: Potatoes, tomatoes, spinach, beets, and winter squash.
  - Legumes: Beans, lentils, and peas.
  - Dairy Products: Milk, yogurt, and cheese.
  - Nuts and Seeds: Almonds, peanuts, and sunflower seeds.
  - Certain Grains: Quinoa and whole wheat products.

2. Choosing Low-Potassium Alternatives

- *Incorporate Low-Potassium Foods:* Focus on including foods that are lower in potassium, such as:
  - Fruits: Apples, berries, grapes, and pears.
  - Vegetables: Zucchini, bell peppers, carrots, cauliflower, and lettuce.
  - Grains: White rice, white bread, and pasta.
  - Proteins: Egg whites, lean meats, and fish (in moderation).

3. Portion Control

- *Monitor Serving Sizes:* Even low-potassium foods can contribute to overall potassium intake if consumed in large quantities. Be mindful of portion sizes to ensure you stay within your potassium limits.

4. Food Preparation Techniques

- *Use Cooking Methods to Reduce Potassium:* Cooking methods can affect the potassium content of certain foods. Techniques include:
  - Leaching: Soaking high-potassium vegetables in water before cooking can help reduce their potassium content.
  - Boiling: Boiling vegetables and discarding the cooking water can significantly lower potassium levels.

5. Read Labels

- *Check Nutritional Information:* Always read food labels to determine potassium content. Many processed and packaged foods can contain hidden sources of potassium in the form of additives or preservatives.

6. Regular Monitoring of Potassium Levels

- *Frequent Blood Tests:* Regular monitoring of potassium levels through blood tests is essential for individuals on a low potassium diet. This helps ensure potassium levels remain within a safe range and allows for dietary adjustments as needed.

7. Consultation with Healthcare Professionals

- *Work with Dietitians and Nephrologists:* Collaborating with healthcare providers, especially registered dietitians and nephrologists, is crucial. They can provide personalized dietary recommendations, meal planning guidance, and education tailored to individual health needs.

8. Stay Hydrated

- *Fluid Intake Considerations:* While potassium management is essential, staying hydrated is also important. However, individuals with kidney disease may need to monitor fluid intake, so consult with a healthcare provider for personalized recommendations.

Following a low potassium diet involves understanding which foods to limit, choosing low-potassium alternatives, and employing effective cooking techniques to manage potassium intake. Regular monitoring and collaboration with healthcare professionals are essential for maintaining health and preventing complications related to potassium levels. With the right knowledge and support, individuals can successfully navigate a low-potassium diet while enjoying a variety of delicious meals.

Cooking Techniques
for Low Potassium Meals

Cooking techniques play a crucial role in managing potassium levels in meals, especially for individuals with chronic kidney disease (CKD) or those requiring potassium management. By employing specific methods, you can reduce the potassium content in certain foods while still enjoying flavorful and nutritious meals. Here are some effective cooking techniques for preparing low-potassium meals:

Leaching
Leaching involves soaking vegetables in water to draw out some of the potassium.

How to Do It:
1. Cut vegetables into smaller pieces.
2. Soak them in a large bowl of water for 2-4 hours, changing the water once or twice.
3. After soaking, rinse the vegetables under cold water before cooking.

Best For: Potatoes, carrots, and other high-potassium vegetables.

Boiling
Boiling vegetables in water can help reduce their potassium content.

How to Do It:
1. Bring a pot of water to a boil.
2. Add the chopped vegetables and boil for 10-15 minutes.
3. Drain the vegetables and discard the cooking water, as it contains leached potassium.

Best For: Potatoes, sweet potatoes, and other starchy vegetables.

Steaming

Steaming cooks vegetables with minimal water, which helps retain nutrients while reducing potassium levels.

How to Do It:
1. Use a steamer basket over a pot of boiling water.
2. Place the vegetables in the basket and cover.
3. Steam for 5-10 minutes until tender.

Best For: Broccoli, zucchini, and bell peppers.

Roasting

Roasting vegetables in the oven can enhance flavor and texture while keeping potassium levels manageable.

How to Do It:
1. Preheat your oven to 400°F (200°C).
2. Toss vegetables with olive oil, herbs, and spices.
3. Spread them on a baking sheet and roast for 20-30 minutes, turning halfway through.

Best For: Carrots, zucchini, and bell peppers.

Sautéing

Sautéing involves cooking vegetables quickly over medium-high heat with a small amount of oil.

How to Do It:
1. Heat olive oil in a skillet.
2. Add chopped vegetables and cook for 5-10 minutes, stirring frequently until tender.

Best For: Bell peppers, spinach, and carrots.

Grilling

Grilling adds a smoky flavor to vegetables and proteins while allowing excess moisture (and some potassium) to drip away.

How to Do It:
1. Preheat the grill to medium heat.
2. Toss vegetables with olive oil, salt, and herbs.
3. Grill on skewers or in a grill basket, turning occasionally until tender.

Best For: Zucchini, bell peppers, and asparagus.

Blanching

Blanching involves briefly boiling vegetables and then quickly cooling them in ice water to stop the cooking process.

How to Do It:
1. Bring a pot of water to a boil.
2. Add the vegetables and cook for 2-3 minutes.
3. Immediately transfer them to a bowl of ice water.
4. Drain and use as desired.

Best For: Green beans, broccoli, and carrots.

Using Low-Potassium Ingredients

- Substitutions: Incorporate low-potassium alternatives into your cooking. For example, use white rice instead of brown rice, or select low-potassium pasta varieties.
- Flavor Enhancements: Use herbs, spices, and citrus juices to enhance flavor without adding potassium.

Utilizing these cooking techniques can significantly help manage potassium intake while still allowing for the preparation of delicious and nutritious meals. By being mindful of how you prepare and cook your food, you can create a varied and satisfying low-potassium diet that supports your health and well-being. Always consult with a healthcare provider or registered dietitian for personalized advice and recommendations tailored to your specific dietary needs.

BREAKFAST
Recipes

Oatmeal with Blueberries

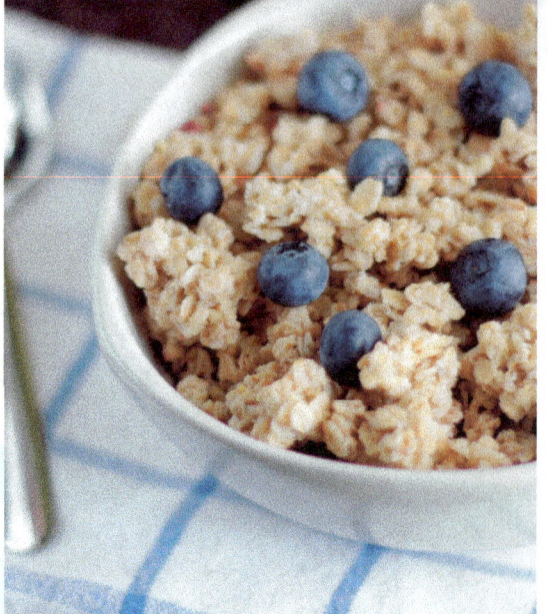

SERVINGS	2
Prep Time	**5 min**
Cook Time	**10 min**
Total Time	**15 min**

Calories	Approximately 150 (without added sweetener)
Protein	Approximately 4g
Fat	Approximately 3g
Carbohydrates	Approximately 28g
Potassium	Approximately 120mg (varies based on ingredients used)

 ## Ingredients

- 1/2 cup rolled oats (low-potassium variety)
- 1 1/2 cups water or low-potassium almond milk
- 1/2 cup fresh blueberries (or frozen, thawed)
- 1 tablespoon maple syrup or honey (optional, for sweetness)
- 1/2 teaspoon cinnamon (optional)
- 1 tablespoon chia seeds (optional, for added nutrition)
- Pinch of salt

ⓘ Instructions

Prepare Oats
- In a medium saucepan, bring the water (or low-potassium almond milk) to a boil. Add a pinch of salt.

Cook Oats
- Stir in the rolled oats and reduce the heat to medium-low. Simmer for about 5-7 minutes, stirring occasionally, until the oats are soft and creamy.

Add Blueberries
- Once the oats are cooked, stir in the fresh or thawed blueberries. If using, add maple syrup or honey and cinnamon for extra flavor. Cook for an additional 1-2 minutes until the blueberries are warmed through.

Serve
- Divide the oatmeal into two bowls. Top with chia seeds if desired. Serve warm and enjoy!

Tips

- **Serving Size:** Adjust the serving size to fit your dietary needs; this recipe is designed to be lower in both protein and potassium.
- **Flavor Boost:** Experiment with adding a dash of vanilla extract or a sprinkle of nutmeg for added flavor without increasing potassium.
- **Customizable:** You can substitute blueberries with lower-potassium fruits such as strawberries or raspberries if desired.

Egg White Omelet with Spinach

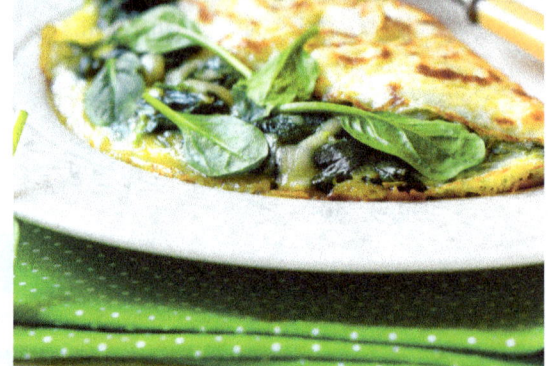

SERVINGS	**2**
Prep Time	**5 min**
Cook Time	**5 min**
Total Time	**10 min**

Calories	Approximately 90 (without cheese)
Protein	Approximately 6g
Fat	Approximately 2g
Carbohydrates	Approximately 6g
Potassium	Approximately 150mg (varies based on ingredients used)

 ## Ingredients

- 4 large egg whites (or 1 cup liquid egg whites)
- 1 cup fresh spinach, chopped
- 1/4 cup bell pepper, diced (optional, for added flavor and color)
- 1/4 cup low-fat cheese (optional, adjust based on potassium preferences)
- Salt and pepper to taste
- Olive oil spray or 1 teaspoon olive oil for cooking

ⓘ Instructions

Prepare Ingredients
- Wash and chop the spinach and bell pepper (if using). Set aside.

Whisk Egg Whites
- In a medium bowl, whisk the egg whites until slightly frothy. Season with a pinch of salt and pepper.

Cook Vegetables
- In a non-stick skillet, lightly spray with olive oil or heat 1 teaspoon of olive oil over medium heat. Add the chopped bell pepper and sauté for 1-2 minutes until slightly softened. Add the spinach and cook for another minute until wilted.

Add Egg Whites
- Pour the whisked egg whites over the sautéed vegetables, tilting the skillet to ensure they spread evenly. Cook for about 2-3 minutes until the edges start to set.

Add Cheese (Optional)
- If using cheese, sprinkle it on top of the omelet now. Continue cooking until the egg whites are fully set and the cheese (if added) is melted, about 1-2 more minutes.

Fold and Serve
- Using a spatula, gently fold the omelet in half and slide it onto a plate. Repeat with the remaining egg whites and vegetables to make a second omelet if desired.

 Tips

- **Cheese Alternatives:** If you want to keep it lower in protein, consider omitting cheese or using a small amount of a low-potassium cheese alternative.
- **Vegetable Variations:** Feel free to include other low-potassium vegetables like zucchini or mushrooms for added texture and flavor.

Low-Potassium Banana Pancakes

SERVINGS	4 pancakes
Prep Time	10 min
Cook Time	10 min
Total Time	20 min

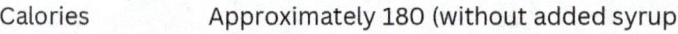

Calories	Approximately 180 (without added syrup)
Protein	Approximately 3g
Fat	Approximately 2g
Carbohydrates	Approximately 36g
Potassium	Approximately 150mg (varies based on ingredients used)

 ## Ingredients

- 1 medium ripe banana (about 4 oz, mashed)
- 1/2 cup all-purpose flour (or a low-potassium flour alternative)
- 1/2 teaspoon baking powder
- 1/4 teaspoon baking soda
- 1/4 teaspoon cinnamon (optional)
- 1/2 cup low-fat milk (or low-potassium almond milk)
- 1 teaspoon vanilla extract (optional)
- Olive oil spray or 1 teaspoon vegetable oil for cooking
- Maple syrup or honey (optional, for serving)

Instructions

Prepare the Batter
- In a mixing bowl, mash the ripe banana until smooth. Add the flour, baking powder, baking soda, cinnamon (if using), milk, and vanilla extract. Mix until just combined; do not overmix.

Heat the Skillet
- Preheat a non-stick skillet or griddle over medium heat. Lightly spray with olive oil or add a teaspoon of vegetable oil.

Cook the Pancakes
- Pour about 1/4 cup of the batter onto the skillet for each pancake. Cook for about 2-3 minutes, or until bubbles form on the surface and the edges look set. Flip and cook for an additional 1-2 minutes until golden brown.

Serve
- Remove the pancakes from the skillet and keep warm while you cook the remaining batter. Serve warm with a drizzle of maple syrup or honey if desired.

Tips

- **Serving Size:** Keep the serving sizes moderate; this recipe is designed to be lower in both protein and potassium.
- **Flavor Options:** Add a sprinkle of nutmeg or use other low-potassium fruits, such as blueberries, instead of bananas for variety.
- **Storage:** Leftover pancakes can be stored in an airtight container in the refrigerator for up to 2 days and reheated in the toaster or microwave.

Yogurt Parfait with Berries

SERVINGS	**2**
Prep Time	**5 min**
Total Time	**5 min**

Calories	Approximately 150 (without added sweetener)
Protein	Approximately 5g
Fat	Approximately 3g
Carbohydrates	Approximately 25g
Potassium	Approximately 150mg (varies based on ingredients used)

 ## Ingredients

- 1 cup low-fat or non-dairy yogurt (check potassium content; coconut yogurt is a good low-potassium option)
- 1/2 cup fresh low-potassium berries (such as strawberries or blueberries)
- 1/4 cup low-potassium granola or crushed rice cereal (check labels for potassium content)
- 1 tablespoon honey or maple syrup (optional, for sweetness)
- 1/2 teaspoon vanilla extract (optional)

ⓘ Instructions

Prepare the Yogurt
- If using plain yogurt, mix in the vanilla extract and honey or maple syrup to sweeten to taste.

Layer the Parfait
- In two serving glasses or bowls, add half of the yogurt as the first layer.

Add Berries
- Layer half of the fresh berries on top of the yogurt.

Add Granola
- Sprinkle half of the granola or crushed rice cereal on top of the berries.

Repeat Layers
- Repeat the layers with the remaining yogurt, berries, and granola.

Serve
- Serve immediately for a refreshing breakfast or snack.

Tips

- **Berry Options:** Use a mix of low-potassium fruits such as strawberries, raspberries, or blackberries to keep potassium levels in check.
- **Yogurt Choice:** Choose a yogurt that is low in potassium and protein, such as coconut or almond yogurt, to suit your dietary needs.
- **Granola Alternatives:** If granola is too high in potassium, consider using crushed rice cakes or a low-potassium cereal instead.
- **Customization:** Feel free to add a sprinkle of cinnamon or nutmeg for extra flavor without added potassium.

Smoothie with Kale and Pear

SERVINGS	**2**
Prep Time	**5 min**
Total Time	**5 min**

Calories	Approximately 150 (without added sweetener or banana)
Protein	Approximately 3g
Fat	Approximately 3g
Carbohydrates	Approximately 30g
Potassium	Approximately 180mg (varies based on ingredients used)

 ## Ingredients

- 1 cup fresh kale, stems removed and chopped (use baby kale for a milder flavor)
- 1 ripe pear, cored and chopped (about 1 medium pear)
- 1/2 banana (optional, adjust based on potassium preference)
- 1 cup low-potassium almond milk (unsweetened) or water
- 1 tablespoon chia seeds (optional, for added nutrition)
- 1 teaspoon honey or maple syrup (optional, for sweetness)
- Ice cubes (optional, for a chilled smoothie)

ⓘ Instructions

Combine Ingredients
- In a blender, add the chopped kale, pear, banana (if using), almond milk (or water), chia seeds (if using), and honey or maple syrup (if desired).

Blend Smoothly
- Blend on high speed until the mixture is smooth and creamy. If you prefer a thicker smoothie, add a few ice cubes and blend again until well combined.

Adjust Consistency
- If the smoothie is too thick, add a little more almond milk or water to reach your desired consistency.

Serve
- Pour the smoothie into two glasses and serve immediately.

Tips

- **Kale Substitution:** If you're looking for an even lower potassium option, consider using spinach or lettuce instead of kale.
- **Sweetness Adjustment:** Adjust the sweetness by adding more or less honey or maple syrup based on your taste preference.
- **Additions:** Enhance the flavor with a dash of cinnamon or a splash of vanilla extract without significantly increasing potassium levels.
- **Storage:** Smoothies are best enjoyed fresh, but if you have leftovers, store them in an airtight container in the refrigerator and consume within 24 hours.

Quinoa Breakfast Bowl

SERVINGS	**2**
Prep Time	**10 min**
Cook Time	**15 min**
Total Time	**25 min**

Calories	Approximately 200 (without added sweetener or yogurt)
Protein	Approximately 6g
Fat	Approximately 3g
Carbohydrates	Approximately 36g
Potassium	Approximately 150mg (varies based on ingredients used)

 ## Ingredients

- 1/2 cup quinoa, rinsed and drained
- 1 cup water or low-potassium almond milk (unsweetened)
- 1/2 medium apple, diced (or pear, for lower potassium)
- 1/4 teaspoon cinnamon (optional)
- 1 tablespoon honey or maple syrup (optional, for sweetness)
- 1 tablespoon chia seeds or sunflower seeds (optional)
- 1/4 cup low-fat yogurt or a low-potassium yogurt alternative (optional)
- Pinch of salt

(i) Instructions

Cook Quinoa
- In a medium saucepan, combine the rinsed quinoa and water (or almond milk) with a pinch of salt. Bring to a boil, then reduce the heat to low, cover, and simmer for about 15 minutes or until the quinoa is fluffy and the liquid is absorbed. Remove from heat and let it sit covered for 5 minutes.

Prepare the Bowl
- Fluff the cooked quinoa with a fork. Divide the quinoa into two bowls.

Add Toppings
- Top each bowl with the diced apple (or pear), a sprinkle of cinnamon, honey or maple syrup (if desired), chia seeds, and yogurt (if using).

Serve
- Enjoy warm or at room temperature as a nutritious breakfast!

Tips

- **Quinoa Alternatives:** For a lower potassium option, consider using a smaller amount of quinoa or substitute it with rice or oats if they fit your dietary needs.
- **Fruit Options:** You can use a variety of low-potassium fruits such as berries or peaches, depending on your preference and availability.
- **Make Ahead:** This quinoa bowl can be prepared ahead of time. Store cooked quinoa in the refrigerator and assemble the bowl in the morning for a quick breakfast.

Savory Breakfast Muffins

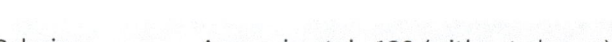

SERVINGS	**12 muffins**
Prep Time	**15 min**
Cook Time	**20 min**
Total Time	**35 min**

Calories	Approximately 120 (without cheese)
Protein	Approximately 3g
Fat	Approximately 4g
Carbohydrates	Approximately 18g
Potassium	Approximately 100mg (varies based on ingredients used)

Ingredients

- 1 1/2 cups all-purpose flour (or a low-potassium flour alternative)
- 1 tablespoon baking powder
- 1/2 teaspoon salt
- 1/4 teaspoon black pepper (optional)
- 1 teaspoon dried herbs (e.g., oregano or thyme)
- 1 cup low-fat milk (or low-potassium almond milk)
- 1/4 cup vegetable oil (or melted coconut oil)
- 2 large egg whites (or 1/4 cup liquid egg whites)
- 1 cup low-potassium vegetables, finely chopped (e.g., zucchini, bell peppers, or spinach)
- 1/2 cup shredded low-fat cheese (optional, adjust based on potassium preferences)

ⓘ Instructions

Preheat the Oven
- Preheat your oven to 375°F (190°C). Line a muffin tin with paper liners or lightly grease it.

Mix Dry Ingredients
- In a large bowl, combine the flour, baking powder, salt, black pepper, and dried herbs. Mix well.

Mix Wet Ingredients
- In another bowl, whisk together the milk, vegetable oil, and egg whites until well combined.

Combine Ingredients
- Pour the wet ingredients into the dry ingredients and stir until just combined. Do not overmix. Gently fold in the chopped vegetables and cheese, if using.

Fill Muffin Tin
- Divide the batter evenly among the muffin cups, filling each about 2/3 full.

Bake
- Bake in the preheated oven for 18-20 minutes or until the muffins are golden brown and a toothpick inserted into the center comes out clean.

Cool and Serve
- Allow the muffins to cool in the pan for a few minutes before transferring to a wire rack to cool completely. Serve warm or at room temperature.

Tips

- **Vegetable Options:** Choose low-potassium vegetables such as zucchini, carrots, or bell peppers. Avoid high-potassium options like tomatoes or potatoes.
- **Storage:** These muffins can be stored in an airtight container in the refrigerator for up to 3 days or frozen for longer storage.

Chia Seed Pudding

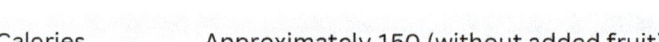

SERVINGS	**2**
Prep Time	**5 min**
Cook Time	**2 min**
Total Time	**5 min**

Calories	Approximately 150 (without added fruit)
Protein	Approximately 4g
Fat	Approximately 6g
Carbohydrates	Approximately 20g
Potassium	Approximately 150mg (varies based on ingredients used)

 ## Ingredients

- 1/4 cup chia seeds
- 1 cup low-potassium almond milk (unsweetened) or low-fat coconut milk
- 1 tablespoon maple syrup or honey (optional, for sweetness)
- 1/2 teaspoon vanilla extract (optional)
- Fresh low-potassium fruit for topping (such as strawberries or blueberries)

(i) Instructions

Combine Ingredients
- In a medium bowl or jar, combine the chia seeds, almond milk (or coconut milk), maple syrup (if using), and vanilla extract (if using).

Mix Well
- Stir the mixture well to ensure that the chia seeds are evenly distributed and not clumped together.

Chill
- Cover the bowl or jar and refrigerate for at least 2 hours or overnight. The chia seeds will absorb the liquid and create a pudding-like consistency.

Serve
- Once thickened, stir the pudding again. Divide it into two bowls or jars. Top with fresh low-potassium fruit, such as sliced strawberries or blueberries, if desired.

Tips

- **Chia Seed Substitution:** If you want to reduce potassium further, consider using a smaller amount of chia seeds, as they can be higher in potassium.
- **Flavor Variations:** Add a pinch of cinnamon or nutmeg for extra flavor without increasing potassium levels.
- **Fruit Options:** Use low-potassium fruits, such as berries, to top your pudding. Avoid high-potassium fruits like bananas or oranges.
- **Storage:** Chia seed pudding can be stored in the refrigerator for up to 3 days. Just stir before serving.

Avocado Toast on Whole Grain Bread

SERVINGS	**2**
Prep Time	**5 min**
Total Time	**5 min**

Calories	Approximately 300 (without additional toppings)
Protein	Approximately 6g
Fat	Approximately 15g
Carbohydrates	Approximately 36g
Potassium	Approximately 300mg (varies based on ingredients used)

 ## Ingredients

- 1 medium avocado (about 4 oz)
- 4 slices of low-potassium whole grain bread (check potassium content on the label)
- 1 tablespoon lemon juice (freshly squeezed)
- Salt and pepper to taste

Optional toppings
- 1/4 teaspoon red pepper flakes (for a kick)
- 1 tablespoon sesame seeds or sunflower seeds (for added crunch)
- Low-potassium vegetables (e.g., cucumber slices or radish slices)

ⓘ Instructions

Toast the Bread
- Toast the whole grain bread slices to your desired crispness.

Prepare the Avocado
- While the bread is toasting, cut the avocado in half, remove the pit, and scoop the flesh into a bowl. Mash it with a fork and mix in the lemon juice. Season with salt and pepper to taste.

Assemble the Toast
- Spread the mashed avocado evenly onto the toasted bread slices.

Add Optional Toppings
- If desired, sprinkle with red pepper flakes, sesame seeds, or sunflower seeds. You can also add low-potassium vegetables like cucumber or radish slices for extra flavor and crunch.

Serve
- Serve immediately and enjoy your nutritious avocado toast!

Tips

- **Bread Selection:** Choose a low-potassium whole grain bread option to keep potassium levels in check. Always check nutritional labels.
- **Avocado Portioning:** If you need to reduce potassium further, consider using half an avocado instead of a whole one.
- **Flavor Enhancements:** Experiment with different herbs, such as dill or cilantro, for added flavor without increasing potassium levels.
- **Make It a Meal:** Pair your avocado toast with a side of low-potassium fruit or a small salad for a complete meal.

Overnight Oats with Almond Milk

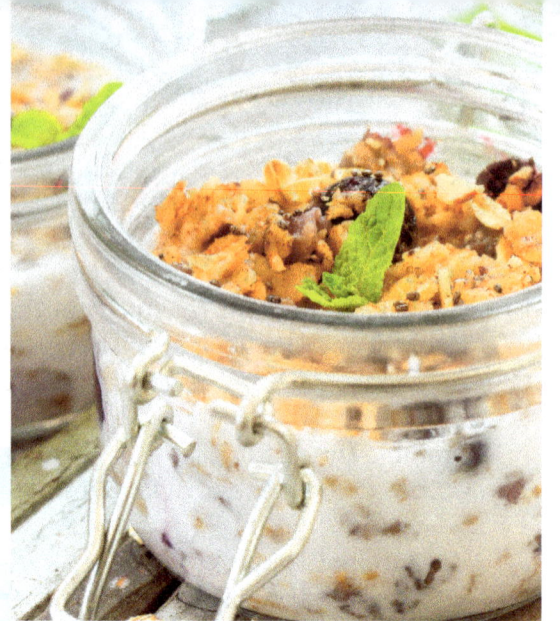

SERVINGS	**2**
Prep Time	**5 min**
Cook Time	**6 min**
Total Time	**5 min**

Calories	Approximately 180 (without added sweetener or toppings)
Protein	Approximately 5g
Fat	Approximately 3g
Carbohydrates	Approximately 32g
Potassium	Approximately 150mg (varies based on ingredients used)

 Ingredients

- 1 cup rolled oats (low-potassium variety)
- 1 1/2 cups unsweetened low-potassium almond milk
- 1 tablespoon maple syrup or honey (optional, for sweetness)
- 1/2 teaspoon vanilla extract (optional)
- 1/2 teaspoon cinnamon (optional)
- 1/2 cup fresh low-potassium fruit for topping (such as strawberries or blueberries)
- 1 tablespoon chia seeds (optional, for added nutrition)

ⓘ Instructions

Combine Ingredients
- In a medium bowl or jar, combine the rolled oats, almond milk, maple syrup (if using), vanilla extract (if using), and cinnamon (if using). Stir well to ensure the oats are fully submerged in the liquid.

Add Chia Seeds
- If using, add the chia seeds to the mixture and stir to combine.

Chill
- Cover the bowl or jar and refrigerate for at least 6 hours or overnight. The oats will absorb the liquid and soften, creating a creamy texture.

Serve
- Once ready to serve, stir the mixture again. Divide the overnight oats into two bowls or jars. Top with fresh low-potassium fruit, such as sliced strawberries, blueberries, or raspberries.

 # Tips

- **Oat Variety:** Ensure that the oats you use are from a low-potassium source. Adjust the amount based on your dietary needs.
- **Fruit Options:** Choose low-potassium fruits for topping to maintain potassium levels. Avoid bananas or high-potassium fruits.
- **Customization:** Feel free to mix in other flavorings or spices, such as nutmeg or shredded coconut, that are low in potassium.
- **Storage:** Overnight oats can be stored in the refrigerator for up to 3 days, making them a convenient option for meal prep.

LUNCH
Recipes

Quinoa Salad with Cucumbers

SERVINGS	**4**
Prep Time	**15 min**
Cook Time	**15 min**
Total Time	**30 min**

Calories	Approximately 180
Protein	Approximately 5g
Fat	Approximately 7g
Carbohydrates	Approximately 25g
Potassium	Approximately 150mg (varies based on ingredients used)

 ## Ingredients

- 1 cup quinoa, rinsed and drained
- 2 cups water or low-potassium vegetable broth
- 1 cup cucumber, diced (peeled if desired)
- 1/2 cup bell pepper, diced (use red or yellow for lower potassium)
- 1/4 cup red onion, finely chopped (optional, adjust based on preference)
- 1 tablespoon olive oil
- 1 tablespoon lemon juice (freshly squeezed)
- 1 teaspoon dried oregano or parsley (optional)
- Salt and pepper to taste

ⓘ Instructions

Cook the Quinoa
- In a medium saucepan, combine the rinsed quinoa and water (or low-potassium vegetable broth). Bring to a boil, then reduce the heat to low, cover, and simmer for about 15 minutes or until the quinoa is fluffy and the liquid is absorbed. Remove from heat and let it sit covered for 5 minutes.

Cool the Quinoa
- After resting, fluff the quinoa with a fork and let it cool for a few minutes.

Prepare the Salad
- In a large bowl, combine the diced cucumber, bell pepper, red onion (if using), and cooled quinoa.

Dress the Salad
- In a small bowl, whisk together the olive oil, lemon juice, oregano (if using), salt, and pepper. Pour the dressing over the quinoa salad and toss gently to combine.

Serve
- Serve immediately or refrigerate for 30 minutes to allow the flavors to meld. This salad can be enjoyed cold or at room temperature.

Tips

- **Quinoa Alternatives:** If you need to reduce potassium further, consider using a smaller amount of quinoa or substitute with low-potassium rice.
- **Custom Vegetables:** Feel free to customize the salad with other low-potassium vegetables like carrots or zucchini for added crunch and nutrition.
- **Meal Prep:** This salad can be made ahead of time and stored in the refrigerator for up to 3 days, making it a great option for meal prep.

Grilled Chicken Salad with Lemon Dressing

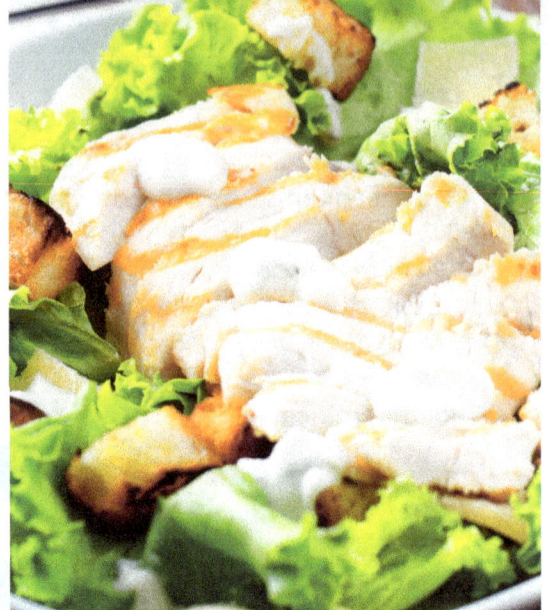

SERVINGS	**4**
Prep Time	**15 min**
Cook Time	**10 min**
Total Time	**25 min**

Calories	Approximately 220 (without feta)
Protein	Approximately 15g (adjust based on chicken portion)
Fat	Approximately 14g
Carbohydrates	Approximately 10g
Potassium	Approximately 250mg (varies based on ingredients)

Ingredients

For the Salad
- 1 boneless, skinless chicken breast (about 4 oz)
- 6 cups mixed salad greens (e.g., romaine, iceberg, and arugula)
- 1/2 cup cherry tomatoes, halved
- 1/2 cucumber, thinly sliced
- 1/4 cup red bell pepper, sliced (optional)
- 1/4 cup feta cheese (optional, adjust based on potassium preferences)
- Salt and pepper to taste
- Olive oil spray (for cooking the chicken)

For the Lemon Dressing
- 2 tablespoons olive oil
- Juice of 1/2 large lemon (about 1 tablespoon)
- 1 teaspoon Dijon mustard (optional)
- 1 teaspoon maple syrup or honey (optional)
- Salt and pepper to taste

ⓘ Instructions

Prepare the Chicken
- Preheat a grill or grill pan over medium heat. Lightly spray the chicken breast with olive oil and season with a pinch of salt and pepper.

Grill the Chicken
- Place the chicken on the grill and cook for about 5-6 minutes on each side, or until the internal temperature reaches 165°F (75°C) and the juices run clear. Remove from heat and let rest for a few minutes.

Slice the Chicken
- Once the chicken has cooled slightly, slice it into thin strips.

For the Salad
Assemble the Salad
- In a large bowl, combine the mixed salad greens, cherry tomatoes, cucumber, and red bell pepper. Add the sliced grilled chicken on top.

For the Dressing
Make the Dressing
- In a small bowl or jar, whisk together the olive oil, lemon juice, Dijon mustard (if using), maple syrup (if desired), salt, and pepper until well combined.

Dress the Salad
- Drizzle the lemon dressing over the salad and toss gently to combine. Top with feta cheese if desired.

Vegetable Wraps with Hummus

SERVINGS	**4**
Prep Time	**10 min**
Total Time	**10 min**

Calories	Approximately 150 (without additional oil)
Protein	Approximately 5g
Fat	Approximately 4g
Carbohydrates	Approximately 25g
Potassium	Approximately 200mg (varies based on ingredients used)

 ## Ingredients

- 4 low-potassium tortillas or wraps (e.g., whole wheat or low-sodium wraps)
- 1/2 cup hummus (store-bought or homemade, check potassium content)
- 1 cup cucumber, sliced
- 1 cup bell peppers, thinly sliced (use red, yellow, or green)
- 1/2 cup shredded carrots (optional, adjust based on potassium preference)
- 1/2 cup spinach or lettuce leaves
- 1/4 cup alfalfa sprouts (optional)
- Salt and pepper to taste
- Optional: 1 tablespoon olive oil or lemon juice for drizzling

ⓘ Instructions

Prepare the Wraps
- Lay out the tortillas or wraps on a clean surface or cutting board.

Spread the Hummus
- Evenly spread about 2 tablespoons of hummus on each tortilla, leaving a small border around the edges.

Add Vegetables
- Layer the sliced cucumber, bell peppers, shredded carrots (if using), spinach or lettuce leaves, and alfalfa sprouts (if using) over the hummus.

Season
- Sprinkle with salt and pepper to taste. If desired, drizzle with olive oil or lemon juice for extra flavor.

Wrap it Up
- Fold in the sides of the tortilla and roll it up tightly from the bottom to the top, securing the fillings inside.

Slice and Serve
- Cut each wrap in half diagonally and serve immediately, or wrap in foil or parchment paper for a portable meal.

Tips

- **Wrap Selection:** Choose low-potassium tortillas or wraps to keep potassium levels in check. Check nutritional labels for potassium content.
- **Vegetable Options:** Customize the wraps with other low-potassium vegetables, such as zucchini or radishes, to suit your taste.
- **Hummus Choices:** If using store-bought hummus, opt for brands that are lower in sodium and potassium. You can also make your own hummus with low-potassium ingredients.
- **Meal Prep:** These wraps can be made ahead of time. Store them in an airtight container in the refrigerator for up to 2 days.

Lentil Soup

SERVINGS	**4**
Prep Time	**10 min**
Cook Time	**30 min**
Total Time	**40 min**

Calories	Approximately 150
Protein	Approximately 8g
Fat	Approximately 4g
Carbohydrates	Approximately 25g
Potassium	Approximately 200mg (varies based on ingredients used)

 ## Ingredients

- 1 cup low-potassium lentils (such as red or yellow lentils)
- 4 cups low-sodium vegetable broth (check potassium content)
- 1 medium carrot, diced
- 1/2 cup celery, diced
- 1/2 medium onion, diced
- 2 cloves garlic, minced
- 1 teaspoon dried thyme or Italian seasoning
- 1 bay leaf
- 1 tablespoon olive oil
- Salt and pepper to taste
- **Optional:** Fresh herbs for garnish (e.g., parsley)

ⓘ Instructions

Prepare Ingredients
- Rinse the lentils under cold water and set aside. Dice the carrot, celery, onion, and mince the garlic.

Sauté Vegetables
- In a large pot, heat the olive oil over medium heat. Add the diced onion, carrot, and celery. Sauté for about 5 minutes, or until the vegetables are softened.

Add Garlic and Seasoning
- Stir in the minced garlic, dried thyme (or Italian seasoning), and bay leaf. Cook for an additional 1-2 minutes until fragrant.

Add Lentils and Broth
- Add the rinsed lentils and vegetable broth to the pot. Bring the mixture to a boil, then reduce the heat to low, cover, and simmer for about 20-25 minutes, or until the lentils are tender.

Season to Taste
- Once the lentils are cooked, remove the bay leaf. Season the soup with salt and pepper to taste. If the soup is too thick, you can add more broth or water to reach your desired consistency.

Serve
- Ladle the soup into bowls and garnish with fresh herbs if desired. Serve warm.

Tips

- **Lentil Choices:** Red and yellow lentils are generally lower in potassium than green or brown lentils, making them a better choice for a low-potassium diet.
- **Vegetable Variations:** You can add other low-potassium vegetables such as zucchini or bell peppers to enhance the flavor and nutrition of the soup.
- **Storage:** This soup can be stored in an airtight container in the refrigerator for up to 3 days. It also freezes well for longer storage.

Turkey and Spinach Stuffed Peppers

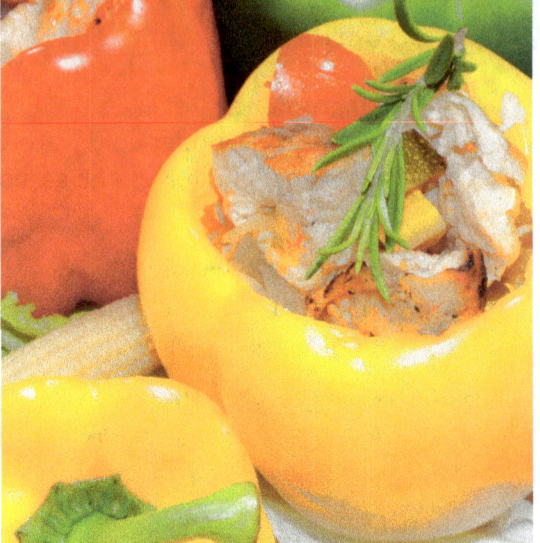

SERVINGS	**4**
Prep Time	**15 min**
Cook Time	**30 min**
Total Time	**45 min**

Calories	Approximately 250 (without cheese)
Protein	Approximately 25g
Fat	Approximately 9g
Carbohydrates	Approximately 20g
Potassium	Approximately 300mg (varies based on ingredients used)

 ## Ingredients

- 4 medium bell peppers (red, yellow, or green)
- 1 pound ground turkey (lean)
- 2 cups fresh spinach, chopped
- 1 cup cooked white rice or quinoa (check potassium content)
- 1/2 cup diced tomatoes (canned or fresh, low-sodium)
- 1/2 teaspoon garlic powder
- 1 teaspoon dried oregano or Italian seasoning
- Salt and pepper to taste
- 1 tablespoon olive oil
- 1/2 cup low-fat cheese (optional, adjust based on potassium preferences)

Preheat the Oven
Preheat your oven to 375°F (190°C).

Prepare the Peppers
Cut the tops off the bell peppers and remove the seeds and membranes. Set aside.

Cook the Turkey
In a large skillet, heat the olive oil over medium heat. Add the ground turkey and cook until browned and fully cooked, about 5-7 minutes. Break it apart with a spoon as it cooks.

Add Vegetables and Seasoning
Once the turkey is cooked, stir in the chopped spinach, diced tomatoes, garlic powder, oregano, salt, and pepper. Cook for an additional 2-3 minutes until the spinach is wilted.

Combine with Rice or Quinoa
In a large bowl, combine the turkey and spinach mixture with the cooked rice or quinoa. Mix well to combine.

Stuff the Peppers
Spoon the turkey and spinach filling into each bell pepper, packing it down lightly. If using, sprinkle the cheese on top of the stuffed peppers.

Bake
Place the stuffed peppers upright in a baking dish. Add a small amount of water to the bottom of the dish to help steam the peppers. Cover with foil and bake for 25 minutes. Remove the foil and bake for an additional 5-10 minutes, or until the peppers are tender and the cheese is melted (if using).

Serve
Remove from the oven and let cool slightly before serving.

Zucchini Noodles with Marinara

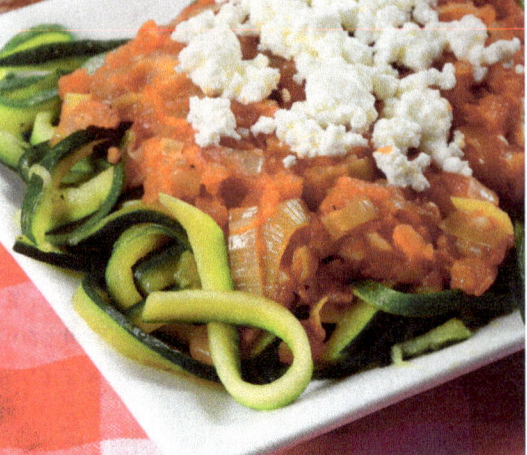

SERVINGS	**2**
Prep Time	**10 min**
Cook Time	**10 min**
Total Time	**20 min**

Calories	Approximately 150 (without cheese)
Protein	Approximately 4g
Fat	Approximately 7g
Carbohydrates	Approximately 20g
Potassium	Approximately 250mg (varies based on ingredients used)

 ## Ingredients

- 2 medium zucchinis (about 1 pound)
- 1 cup low-sodium marinara sauce (check potassium content)
- 1 tablespoon olive oil
- 1 clove garlic, minced (optional)
- 1/2 teaspoon dried Italian seasoning (optional)
- Salt and pepper to taste
- Grated Parmesan cheese (optional, adjust based on potassium preferences)
- Fresh basil or parsley for garnish (optional)

(i) Instructions

Prepare the Zucchini Noodles
- Using a spiralizer or a vegetable peeler, create zucchini noodles (zoodles) from the zucchinis. If using a peeler, make long, thin strips. Set aside.

Sauté Garlic (Optional)
- In a large skillet, heat the olive oil over medium heat. If using garlic, add it to the skillet and sauté for about 1 minute until fragrant (be careful not to burn it).

Cook Zucchini Noodles
- Add the zucchini noodles to the skillet and sauté for about 2-3 minutes, just until they begin to soften. Be careful not to overcook them, as they can become mushy.

Add Marinara Sauce
- Pour the low-sodium marinara sauce over the zucchini noodles. Stir in the dried Italian seasoning, salt, and pepper. Cook for an additional 2-3 minutes until the sauce is heated through.

Serve
- Divide the zucchini noodles and marinara sauce between two plates. If desired, sprinkle with grated Parmesan cheese and garnish with fresh basil or parsley.

Tips

- **Zucchini Size:** Choose medium-sized zucchinis, as they have a lower water content and will hold up better in the dish.
- **Sauce Choices:** Opt for homemade marinara if possible, as store-bought versions can vary in potassium content. Look for low-sodium and low-potassium brands.
- **Additions:** You can add other low-potassium vegetables, such as bell peppers or mushrooms, to the marinara sauce for added flavor and nutrition.
- **Meal Prep:** This dish is best served fresh, but you can prepare the zucchini noodles in advance and store them in the refrigerator for a day.

Chickpea Salad

SERVINGS	**4**
Prep Time	**10 min**
Total Time	**10 min**

Calories	Approximately 160
Protein	Approximately 6g
Fat	Approximately 7g
Carbohydrates	Approximately 20g
Potassium	Approximately 200mg (varies based on ingredients used)

 ## Ingredients

- 1 can (15 oz) low-sodium chickpeas, rinsed and drained (or 1 1/2 cups cooked chickpeas)
- 1 cup cucumber, diced
- 1/2 cup bell pepper, diced (red or yellow for lower potassium)
- 1/4 cup red onion, finely chopped (optional)
- 1/2 cup cherry tomatoes, halved (optional; use sparingly for lower potassium)
- 2 tablespoons olive oil
- 1 tablespoon lemon juice (freshly squeezed)
- 1 teaspoon dried oregano or Italian seasoning
- Salt and pepper to taste
- Fresh parsley or cilantro for garnish (optional)

ⓘ Instructions

Prepare the Ingredients
- Rinse and drain the chickpeas if using canned. Dice the cucumber, bell pepper, and onion (if using). Halve the cherry tomatoes if adding.

Combine Ingredients
- In a large mixing bowl, combine the chickpeas, diced cucumber, bell pepper, red onion, and cherry tomatoes.

Dress the Salad
- In a small bowl, whisk together the olive oil, lemon juice, dried oregano, salt, and pepper. Pour the dressing over the salad and toss gently to combine.

Serve
- Garnish with fresh parsley or cilantro if desired. Serve immediately or refrigerate for 30 minutes to allow the flavors to meld.

Tips

- **Chickpea Alternatives:** If you need to lower potassium further, consider using a smaller amount of chickpeas or substituting with lower-potassium protein sources like cooked quinoa.
- **Vegetable Options:** Feel free to customize the salad with other low-potassium vegetables such as zucchini or radishes if desired.
- **Storage:** This salad can be stored in an airtight container in the refrigerator for up to 3 days.

Baked Sweet Potato with Black Beans

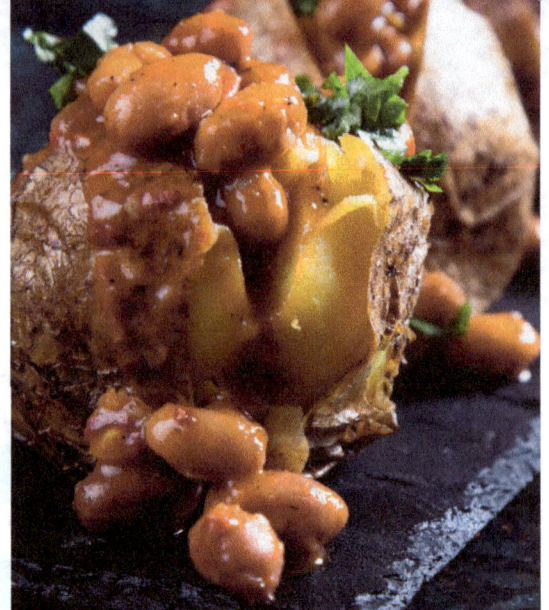

SERVINGS	**2**
Prep Time	**10 min**
Cook Time	**45 min**
Total Time	**55 min**

Calories	Approximately 250 (without Greek yogurt)
Protein	Approximately 8g
Fat	Approximately 5g
Carbohydrates	Approximately 45g
Potassium	Approximately 300mg (varies based on ingredients used)

Ingredients

- 2 medium sweet potatoes (approximately 5 oz each)
- 1 can (15 oz) low-sodium black beans, rinsed and drained
- 1/2 teaspoon cumin (optional)
- 1/2 teaspoon chili powder (optional)
- 1 tablespoon olive oil
- Salt and pepper to taste
- 1/4 cup low-fat Greek yogurt (optional, adjust based on potassium preferences)
- Fresh cilantro or parsley for garnish (optional)

ⓘ Instructions

Preheat the Oven
- Preheat your oven to 400°F (200°C).

Bake the Sweet Potatoes
- Wash the sweet potatoes thoroughly and prick them several times with a fork. Place them on a baking sheet lined with parchment paper or foil. Bake in the preheated oven for about 45 minutes, or until they are tender and easily pierced with a fork.

Prepare the Black Beans
- While the sweet potatoes are baking, heat the black beans in a small saucepan over medium heat. Add cumin, chili powder, salt, and pepper to taste. Stir and cook for about 5 minutes until warmed through.

Assemble the Dish
- Once the sweet potatoes are done baking, remove them from the oven and let them cool slightly. Cut a slit down the center of each sweet potato and gently fluff the insides with a fork.

Top with Black Beans
- Spoon the heated black beans into the center of each sweet potato. If using, top with a dollop of Greek yogurt and garnish with fresh cilantro or parsley.

Serve
- Serve warm and enjoy!

 Tips

- **Sweet Potato Size:** Choose smaller sweet potatoes to help manage potassium levels, as larger ones can be higher in potassium.
- **Bean Alternatives:** If black beans are too high in potassium for your dietary needs, consider using a smaller portion or substituting with a lower potassium legume.

Rice and Vegetable Stir-Fry

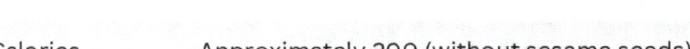

SERVINGS	**4**
Prep Time	**10 min**
Cook Time	**15 min**
Total Time	**25 min**

Calories	Approximately 200 (without sesame seeds)
Protein	Approximately 5g
Fat	Approximately 7g
Carbohydrates	Approximately 30g
Potassium	Approximately 200mg (varies based on ingredients used)

 ## Ingredients

- 2 cups cooked white rice or low-potassium brown rice
- 1 tablespoon olive oil
- 1 cup bell peppers, sliced (red, yellow, or green)
- 1 cup zucchini, sliced
- 1/2 cup carrots, julienned (or sliced thinly)
- 1/2 cup broccoli florets (optional, use sparingly for lower potassium)
- 1/2 cup snap peas or green beans (optional)
- 2 cloves garlic, minced
- 1 tablespoon low-sodium soy sauce (or tamari for gluten-free)
- 1 teaspoon ginger, minced (optional)
- Salt and pepper to taste
- **Optional:** Sesame seeds for garnish

ⓘ Instructions

Prepare the Rice
- If using leftover rice, make sure it is heated through. If cooking fresh rice, prepare according to package instructions.

Heat the Oil
- In a large skillet or wok, heat the olive oil over medium-high heat.

Cook the Vegetables
- Add the minced garlic and ginger (if using) to the skillet and sauté for about 30 seconds until fragrant. Then, add the sliced bell peppers, zucchini, carrots, broccoli, and snap peas (if using). Stir-fry the vegetables for about 5-7 minutes, or until they are tender but still crisp.

Add Rice and Sauce
- Add the cooked rice to the skillet. Pour the low-sodium soy sauce over the rice and vegetables. Toss everything together gently to combine and heat through for another 2-3 minutes.

Season to Taste
- Season with salt and pepper to taste. Adjust the soy sauce if needed.

Serve
- Serve the stir-fry hot, garnished with sesame seeds if desired.

 ## Tips

- **Rice Options:** Use white rice or low-potassium brown rice to keep potassium levels in check. Avoid high-potassium grains like quinoa if necessary.
- **Vegetable Choices:** Feel free to customize the stir-fry with other low-potassium vegetables like bell peppers, asparagus, or cauliflower while avoiding high-potassium options like spinach or tomatoes.
- **Meal Prep:** This stir-fry is great for meal prep and can be stored in an airtight container in the refrigerator for up to 3 days. Reheat in the microwave or on the stove before serving.

Mediterranean Couscous Salad

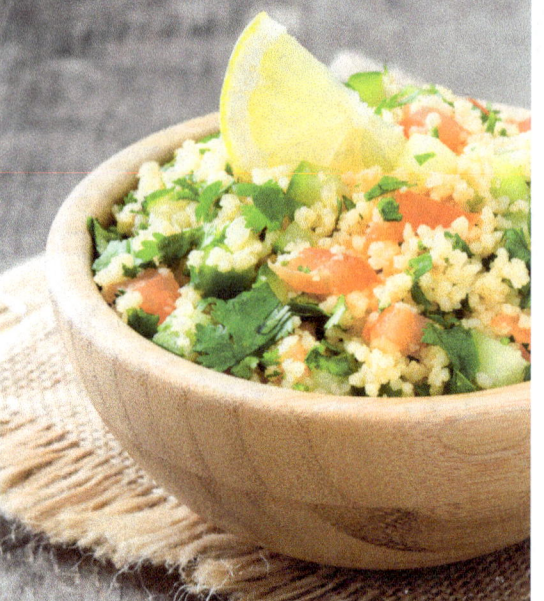

SERVINGS	**4**
Prep Time	**10 min**
Cook Time	**10 min**
Total Time	**20 min**

Calories	Approximately 180 (without optional ingredients)
Protein	Approximately 5g
Fat	Approximately 7g
Carbohydrates	Approximately 25g
Potassium	Approximately 200mg (varies based on ingredients used)

 ## Ingredients

- 1 cup whole wheat couscous (or low-potassium couscous alternative)
- 1 1/4 cups low-sodium vegetable broth or water
- 1 cup cucumber, diced
- 1/2 cup bell pepper, diced (red or yellow for lower potassium)
- 1/4 cup red onion, finely chopped (optional)
- 1/2 cup cherry tomatoes, halved (optional; use sparingly for lower potassium)
- 1/4 cup parsley, finely chopped
- 2 tablespoons olive oil
- 1 tablespoon lemon juice (freshly squeezed)
- 1 teaspoon dried oregano or Italian seasoning
- Salt and pepper to taste

ⓘ Instructions

Prepare the Couscous
- In a medium saucepan, bring the low-sodium vegetable broth or water to a boil. Stir in the couscous, cover, and remove from heat. Let it sit for about 5 minutes until the liquid is absorbed. Fluff with a fork once done.

Prepare the Vegetables
- While the couscous is cooking, dice the cucumber, bell pepper, and onion (if using). Halve the cherry tomatoes if adding.

Combine Ingredients
- In a large mixing bowl, combine the cooked couscous, diced cucumber, bell pepper, red onion, cherry tomatoes, and parsley.

Dress the Salad
- In a small bowl, whisk together the olive oil, lemon juice, oregano, salt, and pepper. Pour the dressing over the couscous salad and toss gently to combine.

Serve
- Serve immediately or refrigerate for about 30 minutes to allow the flavors to meld.

Tips

- **Couscous Alternatives:** If couscous is too high in potassium for your dietary needs, consider using a smaller portion or a lower-potassium grain alternative like rice or quinoa.
- **Vegetable Options:** Adjust the salad with other low-potassium vegetables such as zucchini or carrots to suit your taste.
- **Storage:** This salad can be stored in an airtight container in the refrigerator for up to 3 days, making it a great option for meal prep.

Hi There!

I hope you are enjoying my book so far. I would really appreciate it if you could leave a quick review on Amazon.

Just simply scan the code below using your mobile phone's camera, or you can enter the link below on our web browser.

https://go.renaltracker.com/LowPotassiumCookbook

Thanks a lot!

-Janeth

DINNER
Recipes

Baked Cod with Herbs

SERVINGS	**2**
Prep Time	**10 min**
Cook Time	**15-20 min**
Total Time	**25-30 min**

Calories	Approximately 200
Protein	Approximately 25g
Fat	Approximately 9g
Carbohydrates	Approximately 1g
Potassium	Approximately 300mg (varies based on ingredients used)

 ## Ingredients

- 2 cod fillets (about 4-6 oz each)
- 1 tablespoon olive oil
- 1 tablespoon lemon juice (freshly squeezed)
- 1 teaspoon dried thyme (or other herbs like dill or parsley)
- 1 teaspoon garlic powder
- Salt and pepper to taste

Optional
- Lemon slices for garnish
- Fresh herbs for garnish (e.g., parsley or dill)

ⓘ Instructions

Preheat the Oven
- Preheat your oven to 400°F (200°C).

Prepare the Baking Dish
- Lightly grease a baking dish with olive oil or line it with parchment paper.

Season the Cod
- Place the cod fillets in the baking dish. Drizzle with olive oil and lemon juice. Sprinkle the dried thyme, garlic powder, salt, and pepper over the fillets, ensuring they are evenly coated.

Bake the Cod
- Bake in the preheated oven for 15-20 minutes, or until the fish is opaque and flakes easily with a fork. Baking times may vary depending on the thickness of the fillets.

Serve
- Remove from the oven and let cool slightly. Garnish with lemon slices and fresh herbs if desired. Serve warm with your choice of low-potassium sides.

Tips

- **Cod Alternatives:** If you prefer, you can substitute cod with other low-potassium fish options such as tilapia or haddock.
- **Herb Variations:** Feel free to experiment with different herbs and spices according to your taste preferences, keeping in mind that fresh herbs can enhance flavor without adding potassium.
- **Serving Suggestions:** Pair with low-potassium vegetables like zucchini or a simple salad for a balanced meal.
- **Storage:** Leftover baked cod can be stored in an airtight container in the refrigerator for up to 2 days.

Stir-Fried Tofu with Bell Peppers

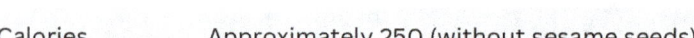

SERVINGS	2
Prep Time	**10 min**
Cook Time	**10-15 min**
Total Time	**20-25 min**

Calories	Approximately 250 (without sesame seeds)
Protein	Approximately 15g
Fat	Approximately 15g
Carbohydrates	Approximately 15g
Potassium	Approximately 250mg (varies based on ingredients used)

 ## Ingredients

- 1 block (14 oz) firm tofu, drained and pressed
- 1 tablespoon olive oil or vegetable oil
- 1 cup bell peppers, sliced (red, yellow, or green)
- 1/2 cup zucchini, sliced (optional)
- 1/2 cup carrots, julienned (optional)
- 2 cloves garlic, minced (optional)
- 1 tablespoon low-sodium soy sauce (or tamari for gluten-free)
- 1 teaspoon ginger, minced (optional)
- Salt and pepper to taste

Optional
- Sesame seeds for garnish

ⓘ Instructions

Prepare the Tofu
- After draining the tofu, press it to remove excess moisture. Cut the tofu into bite-sized cubes.

Heat the Oil
- In a large skillet or wok, heat the olive oil over medium-high heat.

Cook the Tofu
- Add the tofu cubes to the skillet, cooking for about 5-7 minutes, turning occasionally, until they are golden brown on all sides. Remove the tofu from the skillet and set aside.

Stir-Fry the Vegetables
- In the same skillet, add the sliced bell peppers, zucchini, and carrots (if using). Stir-fry for about 3-5 minutes until the vegetables are tender but still crisp. Add the minced garlic and ginger (if using) and stir-fry for an additional minute until fragrant.

Combine Tofu and Sauce
- Return the cooked tofu to the skillet. Add the low-sodium soy sauce, stirring to combine everything. Cook for another 2-3 minutes to heat through and allow the flavors to meld.

Serve
- Season with salt and pepper to taste. Serve hot, garnished with sesame seeds if desired.

Tips

- **Tofu Preparation:** Ensure to press the tofu well to remove excess moisture for better texture and flavor absorption.
- **Vegetable Options:** Feel free to customize the stir-fry with other low-potassium vegetables such as snap peas, broccoli, or mushrooms.
- **Flavor Enhancements:** Adjust the seasoning with herbs or spices that are low in potassium to enhance flavor without compromising dietary needs.

Grilled Salmon with Asparagus

SERVINGS	**2**
Prep Time	**10 min**
Cook Time	**10-15 min**
Total Time	**20-25 min**

Calories	Approximately 300 (without lemon wedges)
Protein	Approximately 30g
Fat	Approximately 18g
Carbohydrates	Approximately 5g
Potassium	Approximately 300mg (varies based on ingredients used)

Ingredients

- 2 salmon fillets (about 4-6 oz each)
- 1 bunch asparagus, trimmed (about 1 lb)
- 1 tablespoon olive oil
- 1 tablespoon lemon juice (freshly squeezed)
- 1 teaspoon dried dill or parsley (optional)
- Salt and pepper to taste

Optional
- Lemon wedges for serving

ⓘ Instructions

Preheat the Grill
- Preheat your grill to medium-high heat.

Prepare the Salmon and Asparagus
- In a small bowl, whisk together the olive oil, lemon juice, dill (if using), salt, and pepper. Brush this mixture onto both sides of the salmon fillets and the asparagus.

Grill the Salmon
- Place the salmon fillets skin-side down on the grill. Grill for about 4-6 minutes on each side, or until the salmon is cooked through and flakes easily with a fork. The internal temperature should reach 145°F (63°C).

Grill the Asparagus
- While grilling the salmon, place the asparagus on the grill. Grill for about 5-7 minutes, turning occasionally, until tender and slightly charred.

Serve
- Remove the salmon and asparagus from the grill. Serve the salmon alongside the grilled asparagus, garnished with lemon wedges if desired.

Tips

- **Salmon Alternatives:** If you prefer, you can substitute salmon with other low-potassium fish options such as cod or tilapia.
- **Asparagus Preparation:** Trim the asparagus to ensure even cooking. You can also use other low-potassium vegetables like zucchini or bell peppers if desired.
- **Marinade Options:** Feel free to experiment with other herbs and spices that are low in potassium to enhance flavor.
- **Storage:** Leftover salmon and asparagus can be stored in an airtight container in the refrigerator for up to 2 days and reheated gently in the microwave or oven.

Chicken with Lemon and Thyme

SERVINGS	4
Prep Time	**10 min**
Cook Time	**30 min**
Total Time	**40 min**

Calories	Approximately 220
Protein	Approximately 30g
Fat	Approximately 10g
Carbohydrates	Approximately 2g
Potassium	Approximately 250mg (varies based on ingredients used)

 ## Ingredients

- 4 boneless, skinless chicken breasts (about 4-6 oz each)
- 2 tablespoons olive oil
- Juice of 1 large lemon (about 2 tablespoons)
- 1 teaspoon dried thyme (or 1 tablespoon fresh thyme)
- 2 cloves garlic, minced
- Salt and pepper to taste

Optional
- Lemon slices for garnish
- Fresh thyme for garnish

ⓘ Instructions

Preheat the Oven
- Preheat your oven to 375°F (190°C).

Prepare the Marinade
- In a small bowl, whisk together the olive oil, lemon juice, dried thyme, minced garlic, salt, and pepper.

Marinate the Chicken
- Place the chicken breasts in a large zip-top bag or shallow dish. Pour the marinade over the chicken, ensuring it is well-coated. Let it marinate for at least 15 minutes (or up to 2 hours in the refrigerator for more flavor).

Bake the Chicken
- Place the marinated chicken breasts in a baking dish. Pour any remaining marinade over the chicken. Bake in the preheated oven for about 25-30 minutes, or until the chicken is cooked through and the internal temperature reaches 165°F (75°C).

Serve
- Remove the chicken from the oven and let it rest for a few minutes. Serve garnished with lemon slices and fresh thyme, if desired.

Tips

- **Chicken Alternatives:** If you prefer, you can substitute chicken breasts with chicken thighs, but ensure they are skinless for a lower fat option.
- **Herb Variations:** Feel free to experiment with other herbs like rosemary or oregano that are low in potassium to enhance flavor.
- **Serving Suggestions:** Pair with low-potassium vegetables like steamed zucchini or a simple green salad for a balanced meal.
- **Storage:** Leftover chicken can be stored in an airtight container in the refrigerator for up to 3 days and reheated gently.

Vegetable Curry

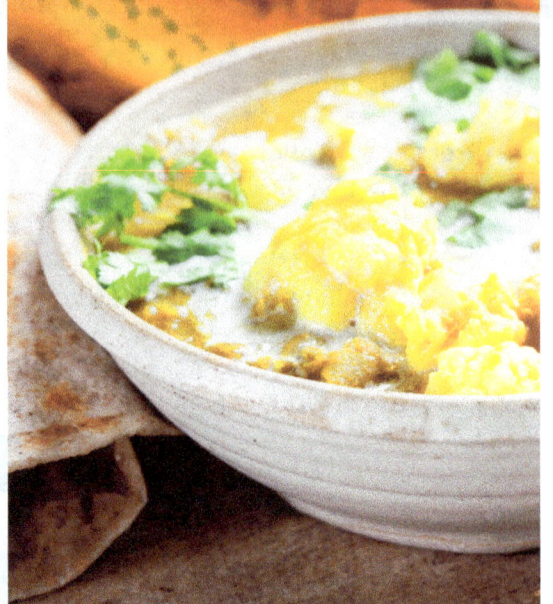

SERVINGS	**4**
Prep Time	**10 min**
Cook Time	**20 min**
Total Time	**30 min**

Calories	Approximately 300 (without rice or quinoa)
Protein	Approximately 6g
Fat	Approximately 20g
Carbohydrates	Approximately 30g
Potassium	Approximately 250mg (varies based on ingredients used)

 ## Ingredients

- 1 tablespoon olive oil
- 1 small onion, diced
- 2 cloves garlic, minced
- 1 tablespoon fresh ginger, minced (or 1 teaspoon ground ginger)
- 1 cup bell peppers, diced (red or yellow for lower potassium)
- 1 cup zucchini, diced
- 1 cup cauliflower florets
- 1 cup carrots, sliced (use sparingly for lower potassium)
- 1 cup low-sodium vegetable broth
- 1 can (14 oz) coconut milk (check potassium content)
- 1 tablespoon curry powder (adjust to taste)
- 1 teaspoon ground cumin
- Salt and pepper to taste

ⓘ Instructions

Heat the Oil
- In a large pot or skillet, heat the olive oil over medium heat. Add the diced onion and sauté for about 3-4 minutes until softened.

Add Garlic and Ginger
- Stir in the minced garlic and ginger, cooking for an additional minute until fragrant.

Add Vegetables
- Add the bell peppers, zucchini, cauliflower, and carrots to the pot. Sauté for about 5-7 minutes until the vegetables start to soften.

Add Spices and Liquids
- Sprinkle in the curry powder and ground cumin, stirring to coat the vegetables. Pour in the vegetable broth and coconut milk, mixing well. Bring the mixture to a gentle simmer.

Cook the Curry
- Reduce the heat to low and let the curry simmer for about 10-15 minutes, or until the vegetables are tender. Stir occasionally to prevent sticking.

Season to Taste
- Season with salt and pepper to taste. If desired, adjust the spice levels by adding more curry powder.

Serve
- Serve the vegetable curry warm, garnished with fresh cilantro if desired. Pair with low-potassium rice or quinoa if using.

 ## Tips

- **Vegetable Choices:** Customize the curry with other low-potassium vegetables such as green beans, asparagus, or eggplant. Avoid high-potassium vegetables like potatoes and tomatoes.
- **Coconut Milk Alternatives:** If coconut milk is too high in potassium, consider using a low-potassium unsweetened almond milk or a low-sodium vegetable broth instead.

Beef and Broccoli Stir-Fry

SERVINGS	**4**
Prep Time	**10 min**
Cook Time	**10 min**
Total Time	**20 min**

Calories	Approximately 250 (without rice)
Protein	Approximately 30g
Fat	Approximately 10g
Carbohydrates	Approximately 10g
Potassium	Approximately 250mg (varies based on ingredients used)

 ## Ingredients

- 1 pound lean beef (such as sirloin or flank steak), thinly sliced
- 2 cups broccoli florets
- 1 tablespoon olive oil
- 2 cloves garlic, minced
- 1 tablespoon low-sodium soy sauce (or tamari for gluten-free)
- 1 teaspoon ginger, minced (optional)
- 1 tablespoon cornstarch (optional, for thickening)
- 1/2 cup low-sodium beef broth or water
- Salt and pepper to taste
- **Optional:** Cooked rice for serving (check potassium content)

Prepare the Beef

- If not already sliced, thinly slice the beef against the grain. This will help keep it tender during cooking.

Heat the Oil

- In a large skillet or wok, heat the olive oil over medium-high heat.

Cook the Beef

- Add the sliced beef to the skillet and stir-fry for about 3-4 minutes, or until browned and cooked through. Remove the beef from the skillet and set aside.

Stir-Fry the Broccoli

- In the same skillet, add the broccoli florets and cook for about 2-3 minutes until they are bright green and slightly tender. If you like your broccoli softer, you can add a splash of water and cover for a minute to steam it.

Add Garlic and Ginger

- Stir in the minced garlic and ginger (if using) and cook for another minute until fragrant.

Combine and Thicken

- Return the cooked beef to the skillet. Add the low-sodium soy sauce and beef broth (or water). If using cornstarch, mix it with a little water to create a slurry and add it to the skillet to thicken the sauce. Stir everything to combine and cook for another 2-3 minutes.

Season to Taste

- Season with salt and pepper to taste.

Serve

- Serve the beef and broccoli stir-fry hot, over a bed of low-potassium rice if desired.

Stuffed Zucchini Boats

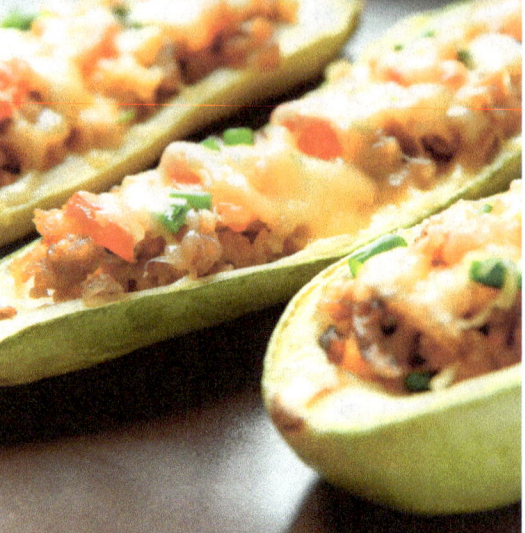

SERVINGS	**4**
Prep Time	**15 min**
Cook Time	**25 min**
Total Time	**40 min**

Calories	Approximately 150 (without cheese)
Protein	Approximately 15g
Fat	Approximately 7g
Carbohydrates	Approximately 10g
Potassium	Approximately 200mg (varies based on ingredients used)

 ## Ingredients

- 2 medium zucchinis
- 1 cup cooked ground turkey or lean ground beef (check potassium content)
- 1/2 cup cooked rice or quinoa (optional; use low-potassium options)
- 1/2 cup diced bell pepper (red or yellow for lower potassium)
- 1/4 cup onion, finely chopped (optional)
- 1 cup low-sodium tomato sauce
- 1 teaspoon Italian seasoning (dried oregano and basil)
- Salt and pepper to taste
- 1/2 cup shredded low-fat cheese (optional, adjust based on potassium preferences)
- Olive oil spray or 1 tablespoon olive oil for drizzling

ⓘ Instructions

Preheat the Oven
- Preheat your oven to 375°F (190°C).

Prepare the Zucchini
- Cut the zucchinis in half lengthwise and scoop out the seeds and some of the flesh to create "boats." Reserve the scooped-out zucchini flesh for the filling. Place the zucchini halves in a baking dish and lightly spray or drizzle with olive oil.

Cook the Filling
- In a skillet over medium heat, sauté the chopped onion and diced bell pepper until softened, about 3-5 minutes. Add the reserved zucchini flesh and cook for an additional 2-3 minutes. Stir in the cooked ground turkey or beef, cooked rice or quinoa (if using), low-sodium tomato sauce, Italian seasoning, salt, and pepper. Cook until heated through.

Stuff the Zucchini Boats
- Spoon the filling mixture into each zucchini boat, packing it down lightly. If using cheese, sprinkle it on top of the stuffed zucchini.

Bake
- Cover the baking dish with foil and bake in the preheated oven for about 20 minutes. Remove the foil and bake for an additional 5-10 minutes, or until the zucchini is tender and the cheese is melted (if using).

Serve
- Remove from the oven and let cool slightly before serving. Enjoy warm!

Tips

- **Zucchini Size:** Choose medium-sized zucchinis to ensure they hold up well during baking and provide a good filling ratio.
- **Meat Alternatives:** You can substitute ground turkey with ground chicken or a plant-based protein that is lower in potassium.

Roast Chicken with Root Vegetables

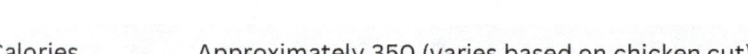

SERVINGS	**4**
Prep Time	**15 min**
Cook Time	**1 hr**
Total Time	**1 hr 15 min**

Calories	Approximately 350 (varies based on chicken cut)
Protein	Approximately 25g
Fat	Approximately 20g
Carbohydrates	Approximately 20g
Potassium	Approximately 400mg (varies based on ingredients used)

 ## Ingredients

For the Chicken
- 4 bone-in, skin-on chicken thighs or breasts (about 4-6 oz each)
- 2 tablespoons olive oil
- 1 tablespoon fresh lemon juice
- 1 teaspoon dried thyme or rosemary
- 1 teaspoon garlic powder
- Salt and pepper to taste

For the Vegetables
- 2 medium carrots, peeled and cut into chunks
- 1 medium parsnip, peeled and cut into chunks (optional, as parsnips are higher in potassium)
- 1 medium turnip, peeled and cut into chunks

- 1 cup rutabaga, peeled and cut into chunks
- 1/2 teaspoon dried thyme or rosemary
- 1 tablespoon olive oil
- Salt and pepper to taste

ⓘ Instructions

Preheat the Oven
- Preheat your oven to 400°F (200°C).

Prepare the Chicken
- In a small bowl, combine the olive oil, lemon juice, dried thyme, garlic powder, salt, and pepper. Rub this mixture all over the chicken pieces.

Prepare the Vegetables
- In a separate bowl, toss the carrots, parsnip (if using), turnip, and rutabaga with olive oil, dried thyme, salt, and pepper until evenly coated.

Arrange in Baking Dish
- Place the chicken pieces in a roasting pan or large baking dish. Surround the chicken with the prepared root vegetables.

Roast
- Roast in the preheated oven for about 1 hour, or until the chicken is cooked through and the internal temperature reaches 165°F (75°C), and the vegetables are tender. Stir the vegetables halfway through the cooking time to ensure even roasting.

Serve
- Remove the roasting pan from the oven and let the chicken rest for a few minutes before serving. Serve the chicken alongside the roasted root vegetables.

Tips

- **Chicken Options:** You can use skinless chicken thighs or breasts for a lower-fat option, but skin adds flavor during roasting.

Pasta Primavera

SERVINGS	**4**
Prep Time	**10 min**
Cook Time	**15 min**
Total Time	**25 min**

Calories	Approximately 250 (without cheese)
Protein	Approximately 8g
Fat	Approximately 8g
Carbohydrates	Approximately 38g
Potassium	Approximately 200mg (varies based on ingredients used)

 ## Ingredients

- 8 oz low-potassium pasta (e.g., whole wheat or gluten-free)
- 2 tablespoons olive oil
- 1 cup bell peppers, sliced (red or yellow for lower potassium)
- 1 cup zucchini, sliced
- 1/2 cup carrots, julienned (use sparingly for lower potassium)
- 1 cup broccoli florets (optional, use sparingly)
- 2 cloves garlic, minced
- 1 teaspoon dried Italian seasoning (or fresh herbs like basil or parsley)
- Salt and pepper to taste
- 1/4 cup grated Parmesan cheese (optional, adjust based on potassium preferences)

ⓘ Instructions

Cook the Pasta
- In a large pot of boiling salted water, cook the low-potassium pasta according to package instructions until al dente. Reserve 1/2 cup of pasta water, then drain the pasta and set aside.

Sauté the Vegetables
- In a large skillet, heat the olive oil over medium heat. Add the minced garlic and sauté for about 30 seconds until fragrant.

Add Vegetables
- Add the bell peppers, zucchini, carrots, and broccoli (if using) to the skillet. Sauté the vegetables for about 5-7 minutes, or until they are tender but still crisp.

Combine Pasta and Vegetables
- Add the cooked pasta to the skillet with the vegetables. Pour in the reserved pasta water gradually, and sprinkle with Italian seasoning, salt, and pepper. Toss everything together to combine and heat through.

Serve
- If desired, sprinkle with grated Parmesan cheese and garnish with fresh basil or parsley before serving. Serve warm.

Tips

- **Pasta Selection:** Choose low-potassium pasta options to keep potassium levels in check. Whole wheat or gluten-free pastas are good choices.
- **Vegetable Options:** Customize the primavera with other low-potassium vegetables like asparagus, green beans, or spinach, avoiding high-potassium options like tomatoes.
- **Serving Suggestions:** Serve with a side salad of low-potassium greens for a complete meal.
- **Storage:** Leftover pasta primavera can be stored in an airtight container in the refrigerator for up to 3 days and reheated in the microwave or on the stovetop.

Low-Potassium Chili

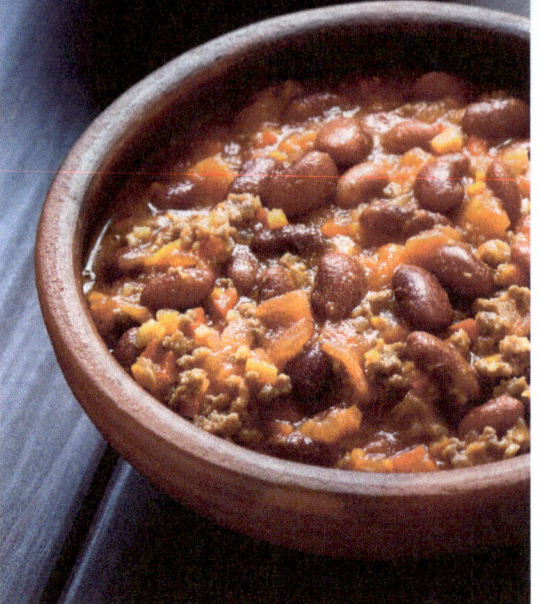

SERVINGS	**4**
Prep Time	**10 min**
Cook Time	**30 min**
Total Time	**40 min**

Calories	Approximately 250 (without beans)
Protein	Approximately 20g
Fat	Approximately 10g
Carbohydrates	Approximately 15g
Potassium	Approximately 250mg (varies based on ingredients used)

 ## Ingredients

- 1 pound ground turkey or lean ground beef (check potassium content)
- 1 tablespoon olive oil
- 1 medium onion, diced
- 2 cloves garlic, minced
- 1 cup bell peppers, diced (red or yellow for lower potassium)
- 1 cup zucchini, diced
- 1 can (15 oz) low-sodium kidney beans or black beans, rinsed and drained (optional, check potassium content)
- 1 can (15 oz) low-sodium diced tomatoes (or fresh tomatoes, peeled and chopped)
- 1 tablespoon chili powder
- 1 teaspoon ground cumin

- 1 teaspoon ground cumin
- 1 teaspoon dried oregano
- 1/2 teaspoon paprika (optional)
- Salt and pepper to taste
- 1 cup low-sodium vegetable broth or water (adjust for desired consistency)

ⓘ Instructions

Cook the Meat
- In a large pot or Dutch oven, heat the olive oil over medium heat. Add the ground turkey or beef and cook until browned, about 5-7 minutes. Drain any excess fat if necessary.

Sauté the Vegetables
- Add the diced onion, minced garlic, and bell peppers to the pot. Sauté for about 3-4 minutes until the vegetables are softened.

Add Zucchini and Spices
- Stir in the diced zucchini, chili powder, ground cumin, dried oregano, paprika (if using), salt, and pepper. Cook for an additional 2 minutes until the spices are fragrant.

Combine Ingredients
- Add the low-sodium kidney beans (if using), diced tomatoes, and low-sodium vegetable broth or water to the pot. Stir well to combine.

Simmer
- Bring the chili to a gentle simmer. Reduce the heat to low and let it cook uncovered for about 20 minutes, stirring occasionally. If the chili is too thick, add more broth or water to reach your desired consistency.

Serve
- Taste and adjust seasoning if needed. Serve warm, garnished with fresh herbs if desired.

SNACK AND DESSERT

Recipes

Hummus with Carrot Sticks

SERVINGS	**4**
Prep Time	**15 min**
Total Time	**15 min**

Calories	Approximately 150 (without tahini)
Protein	Approximately 5g
Fat	Approximately 8g
Carbohydrates	Approximately 15g
Potassium	Approximately 200mg (varies based on ingredients used)

Ingredients

For the Hummus
- 1 can (15 oz) low-sodium chickpeas, rinsed and drained (or about 1 1/2 cups cooked chickpeas)
- 2 tablespoons tahini (optional, check potassium content)
- 2 tablespoons olive oil
- 2 tablespoons lemon juice (freshly squeezed)
- 1 clove garlic, minced (optional)
- Salt to taste
- Water (as needed for desired consistency)

Optional
- 1/2 teaspoon ground cumin or paprika for flavor
- For the Carrot Sticks:
- 4 medium carrots, peeled and cut into sticks

ⓘ Instructions

Prepare the Hummus
Blend Ingredients
- In a food processor, combine the rinsed chickpeas, tahini (if using), olive oil, lemon juice, minced garlic (if using), and salt. Blend until smooth.

Adjust Consistency
- If the hummus is too thick, add water a tablespoon at a time until you reach your desired consistency. Blend again until smooth.

Season
- Taste the hummus and adjust the seasoning. If desired, add ground cumin or paprika for extra flavor and blend until combined.

Prepare the Carrot Sticks
Cut Carrots
- Peel the carrots and cut them into sticks or rounds for dipping.

Serve
Presentation
- Serve the hummus in a bowl with the carrot sticks arranged around it for dipping. Enjoy as a healthy snack or appetizer!

Tips

- **Chickpea Alternatives:** If chickpeas are too high in potassium for your dietary needs, consider using a smaller portion or a lower-potassium bean alternative.
- **Flavor Variations:** Experiment with adding herbs like parsley or spices like turmeric for additional flavor without increasing potassium.
- **Storage:** Store any leftover hummus in an airtight container in the refrigerator for up to 4 days. Serve with additional fresh vegetable sticks or crackers.

Rice Cakes with Almond Butter

SERVINGS	2
Prep Time	**5 min**
Total Time	**5 min**

Calories	Approximately 300 (without additional toppings)
Protein	Approximately 8g
Fat	Approximately 18g
Carbohydrates	Approximately 30g
Potassium	Approximately 200mg (varies based on ingredients used)

 ## Ingredients

- 4 plain rice cakes (check potassium content)
- 4 tablespoons almond butter (check for low-sodium options)
- 1 tablespoon honey or maple syrup (optional, for sweetness)
- 1/2 banana, sliced (optional, use sparingly due to potassium content)
- **Optional toppings:** cinnamon, chia seeds, or a few low-potassium berries (such as strawberries or blueberries)

ⓘ Instructions

Prepare the Rice Cakes
- Place the rice cakes on a clean surface or plate.

Spread Almond Butter
- Evenly spread 1 tablespoon of almond butter on each rice cake.

Add Sweetener (Optional)
- If desired, drizzle honey or maple syrup over the almond butter for added sweetness.

Top with Fruit (Optional)
- If using, add a few slices of banana on top of the almond butter. You can also sprinkle with cinnamon or chia seeds for added flavor and nutrition.

Serve
- Enjoy immediately as a quick snack or light meal!

 ## Tips

- **Rice Cake Selection:** Choose plain rice cakes that are low in sodium and potassium. Avoid flavored varieties that may contain additives.
- **Nut Butter Alternatives:** If almond butter is too high in potassium for your needs, consider using sunflower seed butter or a low-potassium nut butter alternative.
- **Fruit Options:** If bananas are too high in potassium for your diet, consider topping with low-potassium fruits such as strawberries or blueberries in moderation.
- **Storage:** Rice cakes are best enjoyed fresh, but you can prepare them ahead of time. Just wait to add toppings until you're ready to eat to prevent sogginess.

Low-Potassium Fruit Salad

SERVINGS	**4**
Prep Time	**10 min**
Total Time	**10 min**

Calories	Approximately 100
Protein	Approximately 1g
Fat	Approximately 0g
Carbohydrates	Approximately 25g
Potassium	Approximately 150mg (varies based on ingredients used)

 ## Ingredients

- 1 cup strawberries, hulled and sliced
- 1 cup blueberries
- 1 cup raspberries
- 1 medium apple, diced (choose a variety lower in potassium, such as Fuji or Gala)
- 1/2 cup pineapple chunks (fresh or canned in juice, drained)
- 1 tablespoon honey or maple syrup (optional, for sweetness)
- 1 tablespoon fresh lemon juice (optional, to enhance flavor and prevent browning)
- **Optional:** Fresh mint leaves for garnish

ⓘ Instructions

Prepare the Fruit
- In a large mixing bowl, combine the sliced strawberries, blueberries, raspberries, diced apple, and pineapple chunks.

Add Sweetener and Lemon Juice
- If desired, drizzle honey or maple syrup over the fruit mixture and add fresh lemon juice. Toss gently to combine.

Serve
- Divide the fruit salad into individual servings. Garnish with fresh mint leaves if desired. Enjoy immediately or chill for a short time before serving.

Tips

- **Fruit Selection:** Choose fruits that are lower in potassium. Avoid high-potassium fruits such as bananas, oranges, and avocados.
- **Customization:** Feel free to adjust the fruit selection based on seasonal availability and personal preference while keeping potassium levels in mind.
- **Storage:** This fruit salad is best enjoyed fresh but can be stored in an airtight container in the refrigerator for up to 2 days. If storing, add the lemon juice to help prevent browning of the apple.

Coconut Macaroons

SERVINGS	**12**
Prep Time	**15 min**
Cook Time	**20 min**
Total Time	**35 min**

Calories	Approximately 90 (without chocolate)
Protein	Approximately 1g
Fat	Approximately 5g
Carbohydrates	Approximately 10g
Potassium	Approximately 50mg (varies based on ingredients used)

 ## Ingredients

- 2 1/2 cups unsweetened shredded coconut
- 1/2 cup granulated sugar (or a sugar substitute suitable for baking)
- 2 large egg whites
- 1 teaspoon vanilla extract
- 1/4 teaspoon almond extract (optional)
- Pinch of salt
- **Optional:** 1/2 cup dark chocolate chips (check potassium content) for drizzling

ⓘ Instructions

Preheat the Oven
- Preheat your oven to 325°F (160°C). Line a baking sheet with parchment paper.

Mix the Ingredients
- In a large mixing bowl, combine the unsweetened shredded coconut, sugar, egg whites, vanilla extract, almond extract (if using), and a pinch of salt. Mix until well combined.

Form the Macaroons
- Using your hands or a small cookie scoop, form small mounds of the coconut mixture and place them onto the prepared baking sheet, spacing them about 1 inch apart.

Bake
- Bake in the preheated oven for about 20 minutes, or until the macaroons are golden brown on top.

Cool
- Remove from the oven and let the macaroons cool on the baking sheet for a few minutes before transferring them to a wire rack to cool completely.

Chocolate Drizzle (Optional)
- If desired, melt dark chocolate chips in a microwave-safe bowl in 30-second intervals until smooth. Drizzle over the cooled macaroons for added flavor.

Tips

- **Coconut Type:** Make sure to use unsweetened shredded coconut to keep sugar levels lower. Sweetened coconut can increase both sugar and potassium levels.
- **Storage:** Store macaroons in an airtight container at room temperature for up to 5 days. They can also be frozen for longer storage.
- **Customization:** Feel free to experiment with flavors by adding a pinch of cinnamon or using different extracts.

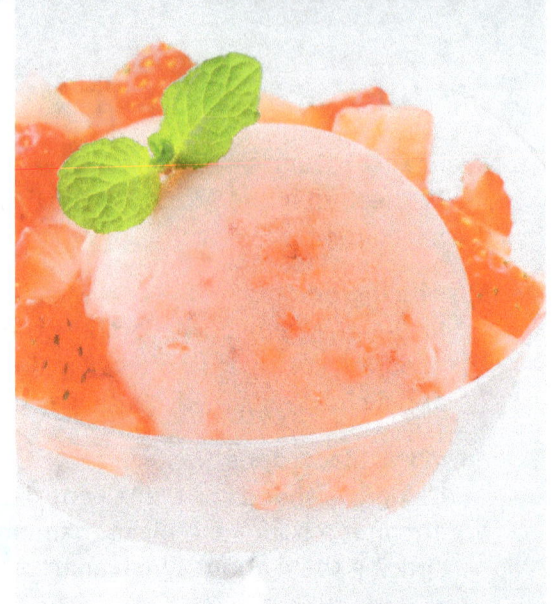

Berry Sorbet

SERVINGS	4
Prep Time	**10 min**
Total Time	**10 min**

Calories	Approximately 80 (without additional sugar)
Protein	Approximately 1g
Fat	Approximately 0g
Carbohydrates	Approximately 20g
Potassium	Approximately 150mg (varies based on ingredients used)

 ## Ingredients

- 2 cups mixed low-potassium berries (such as strawberries, blueberries, and raspberries)
- 1/2 cup granulated sugar (or a sugar substitute suitable for baking)
- 1 tablespoon lemon juice (freshly squeezed)
- 1 teaspoon vanilla extract (optional)
- 1/2 cup water (as needed)

ⓘ Instructions

Prepare the Berries
- If using fresh berries, wash them thoroughly. If using frozen berries, allow them to thaw slightly for easier blending.

Blend the Ingredients
- In a blender or food processor, combine the mixed berries, sugar, lemon juice, and vanilla extract (if using). Blend until smooth. If the mixture is too thick, add water a tablespoon at a time until you reach your desired consistency.

Taste and Adjust
- Taste the mixture and adjust sweetness if necessary by adding more sugar or a sugar substitute.

Freeze the Mixture
- Pour the berry mixture into a shallow container and spread it out evenly. Cover with a lid or plastic wrap and freeze for at least 2-4 hours, or until completely firm.

Serve
- Once the sorbet is frozen, remove it from the freezer and let it sit for a few minutes to soften slightly. Scoop the sorbet into bowls or cups and serve immediately.

Tips

- **Berry Selection:** Choose a mix of low-potassium berries to keep potassium levels in check. Avoid high-potassium fruits like bananas or oranges.
- **Sweetener Options:** If you prefer a lower-calorie option, consider using a sugar substitute that measures like sugar.
- **Storage:** Store any leftover sorbet in an airtight container in the freezer for up to 2 weeks. Allow it to soften slightly before serving if it becomes too hard.
- **Customization:** Feel free to mix different low-potassium fruits or add herbs like mint for a refreshing twist.

Muffins with Applesauce

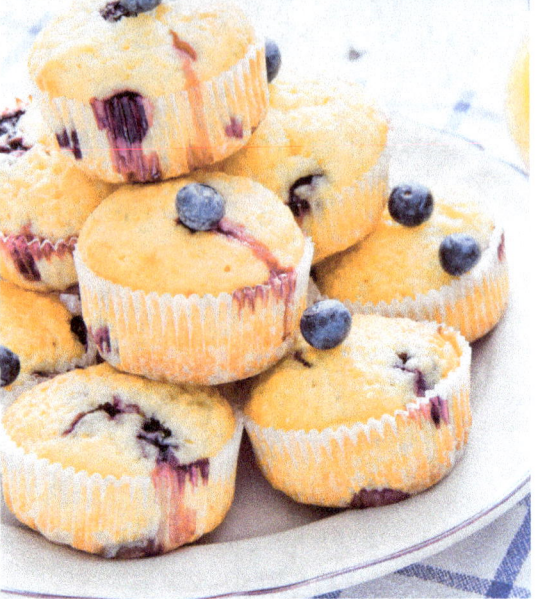

SERVINGS	**12**
Prep Time	**15 min**
Cook Time	**20 min**
Total Time	**35 min**

Calories	Approximately 130 (without added fruits or nuts)
Protein	Approximately 2g
Fat	Approximately 4g
Carbohydrates	Approximately 22g
Potassium	Approximately 120mg (varies based on ingredients used)

 ## Ingredients

- 1 1/2 cups all-purpose flour (or a low-potassium flour alternative)
- 1/2 cup granulated sugar (or a sugar substitute suitable for baking)
- 1 teaspoon baking powder
- 1 teaspoon baking soda
- 1/2 teaspoon salt
- 1 teaspoon cinnamon (optional)
- 1/2 cup unsweetened applesauce
- 1/2 cup low-fat milk (or low-potassium almond milk)
- 1/4 cup vegetable oil or melted coconut oil
- 1 teaspoon vanilla extract
- **Optional:** 1/2 cup low-potassium fruits (such as blueberries or raspberries) or nuts (if within potassium limits)

ⓘ Instructions

Preheat the Oven
- Preheat your oven to 350°F (175°C). Line a muffin tin with paper liners or lightly grease it.

Mix Dry Ingredients
- In a large mixing bowl, whisk together the flour, sugar, baking powder, baking soda, salt, and cinnamon (if using).

Combine Wet Ingredients
- In a separate bowl, mix the applesauce, low-fat milk, oil, and vanilla extract until well combined.

Combine Ingredients
- Pour the wet ingredients into the dry ingredients and stir until just combined. If desired, fold in the low-potassium fruits or nuts.

Fill Muffin Tin
- Divide the batter evenly among the prepared muffin cups, filling each about 2/3 full.

Bake
- Bake in the preheated oven for 20-25 minutes, or until a toothpick inserted into the center comes out clean.

Cool
- Allow the muffins to cool in the tin for a few minutes before transferring them to a wire rack to cool completely.

Tips

- **Flour Selection:** Use low-potassium flour alternatives if necessary, such as a blend of all-purpose and almond flour.
- **Fruit Options:** Opt for low-potassium fruits like blueberries or raspberries. Avoid high-potassium fruits like bananas and dried fruits.
- **Storage:** Store muffins in an airtight container at room temperature for up to 3 days or freeze for longer storage.

Energy Bites with Oats and Honey

SERVINGS	**12**
Prep Time	**10 min**
Total Time	**10 min**

Calories	Approximately 100
Protein	Approximately 3g
Fat	Approximately 5g
Carbohydrates	Approximately 12g
Potassium	Approximately 70mg (varies based on ingredients used)

 ## Ingredients

- 1 cup rolled oats (low-potassium variety)
- 1/2 cup natural almond butter or peanut butter (check potassium content)
- 1/3 cup honey or maple syrup
- 1/4 cup mini chocolate chips (optional, check for low-potassium options)
- 1/4 cup ground flaxseed (optional, for added nutrition)
- 1 teaspoon vanilla extract
- Pinch of salt
- **Optional:** 1/4 cup shredded coconut (unsweetened, check potassium content)

ⓘ Instructions

Combine Ingredients
- In a large mixing bowl, combine the rolled oats, almond butter (or peanut butter), honey (or maple syrup), mini chocolate chips (if using), ground flaxseed (if using), vanilla extract, and a pinch of salt. Mix well until all ingredients are thoroughly combined.

Form the Bites
- Using your hands, scoop out about 1 tablespoon of the mixture and roll it into a ball. Repeat until all the mixture is used.

Chill
- Place the energy bites on a baking sheet lined with parchment paper. Refrigerate for at least 30 minutes to help them firm up.

Serve
- Once chilled, the energy bites are ready to enjoy! Store leftovers in an airtight container in the refrigerator for up to one week.

 ## Tips

- **Oat Selection:** Make sure to use rolled oats that are lower in potassium, as some varieties can vary.
- **Nut Butter Alternatives:** If almond or peanut butter is too high in potassium, consider using sunflower seed butter or a low-potassium nut butter alternative.
- **Sweetener Options:** Adjust sweetness based on your preference by adding more or less honey or maple syrup.
- **Customization:** Feel free to add other low-potassium ingredients such as chia seeds or different types of unsweetened shredded coconut for variety.

Chocolate Avocado Mousse

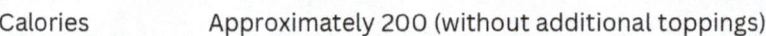

SERVINGS	**2-4**
Prep Time	**10 min**
Total Time	**10 min**

Calories	Approximately 200 (without additional toppings)
Protein	Approximately 3g
Fat	Approximately 12g
Carbohydrates	Approximately 24g
Potassium	Approximately 300mg (varies based on ingredients used)

 ## Ingredients

- 1 ripe avocado (about 4 oz)
- 1/4 cup unsweetened cocoa powder
- 1/4 cup maple syrup or honey (adjust based on sweetness preference)
- 1/4 cup low-fat milk (or low-potassium almond milk)
- 1 teaspoon vanilla extract
- Pinch of salt
- **Optional toppings:** fresh berries (like strawberries or blueberries), chopped nuts (if within potassium limits), or a dollop of whipped cream

ⓘ Instructions

Blend Ingredients
- In a blender or food processor, combine the ripe avocado, cocoa powder, maple syrup or honey, low-fat milk (or almond milk), vanilla extract, and a pinch of salt. Blend until smooth and creamy.

Adjust Consistency
- If the mousse is too thick, add a little more milk to reach your desired consistency, blending again until smooth.

Taste and Adjust
- Taste the mousse and adjust sweetness if needed by adding more maple syrup or honey.

Chill
- Transfer the mousse to serving bowls or cups. Chill in the refrigerator for at least 30 minutes to help it set and enhance the flavors.

Serve
- Once chilled, serve the mousse topped with fresh berries, chopped nuts, or a dollop of whipped cream if desired.

 ## Tips

- **Avocado Selection:** Use ripe avocados for the best flavor and creaminess. They should yield slightly when pressed.
- **Sweetener Options:** Adjust the sweetness according to your taste preference. You can also use a sugar substitute if desired.
- **Storage:** Leftover mousse can be stored in an airtight container in the refrigerator for up to 2 days. Stir before serving if it thickens.

Homemade Granola Bars

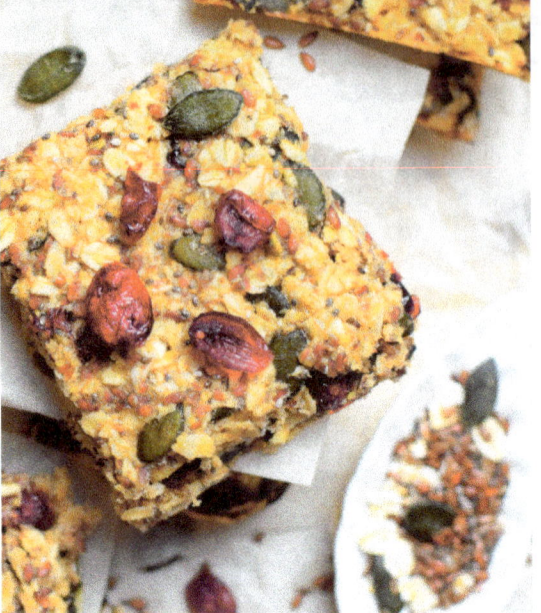

SERVINGS	**10**
Prep Time	**10 min**
Cook Time	**20 min**
Total Time	**30 min**

Calories	Approximately 150 (without chocolate)
Protein	Approximately 4g
Fat	Approximately 7g
Carbohydrates	Approximately 20g
Potassium	Approximately 100mg (varies based on ingredients used)

 ## Ingredients

- 2 cups rolled oats (low-potassium variety)
- 1/2 cup unsweetened nut butter (such as almond butter or sunflower seed butter; check potassium content)
- 1/3 cup honey or maple syrup
- 1/2 cup low-potassium nuts (e.g., walnuts, pecans, or sunflower seeds; check potassium content)
- 1/4 cup dried fruit, chopped (such as cranberries or blueberries; use sparingly due to potassium content)
- 1/4 teaspoon cinnamon (optional)
- Pinch of salt
- **Optional:** 1/4 cup dark chocolate chips (check potassium content) for drizzling

ⓘ Instructions

Preheat the Oven
- Preheat your oven to 350°F (175°C). Line an 8-inch square baking dish with parchment paper, leaving some overhang for easy removal.

Mix Ingredients
- In a large mixing bowl, combine the rolled oats, nut butter, honey (or maple syrup), chopped nuts, dried fruit, cinnamon (if using), and a pinch of salt. Mix well until all ingredients are evenly combined.

Press into Baking Dish
- Transfer the mixture to the prepared baking dish. Using a spatula or your hands, press the mixture firmly into an even layer.

Bake
- Bake in the preheated oven for about 20 minutes, or until the edges are golden brown. Remove from the oven and let it cool in the baking dish for about 10 minutes.

Cut into Bars
- Once cooled, lift the granola mixture out of the baking dish using the parchment paper overhang. Place it on a cutting board and cut into bars or squares.

Optional Chocolate Drizzle
- If desired, melt dark chocolate chips in a microwave-safe bowl in 30-second intervals until smooth. Drizzle over the cooled granola bars.

Store
- Store the granola bars in an airtight container at room temperature for up to 1 week or in the refrigerator for up to 2 weeks.

 ## Tips

- **Nut Butter Choices:** Choose a nut butter that fits your dietary needs. Sunflower seed butter is a great nut-free option.
- **Dried Fruit:** Use dried fruits in moderation, as they can be higher in potassium. Consider using fresh berries instead if desired.

Yogurt with Honey and Nuts

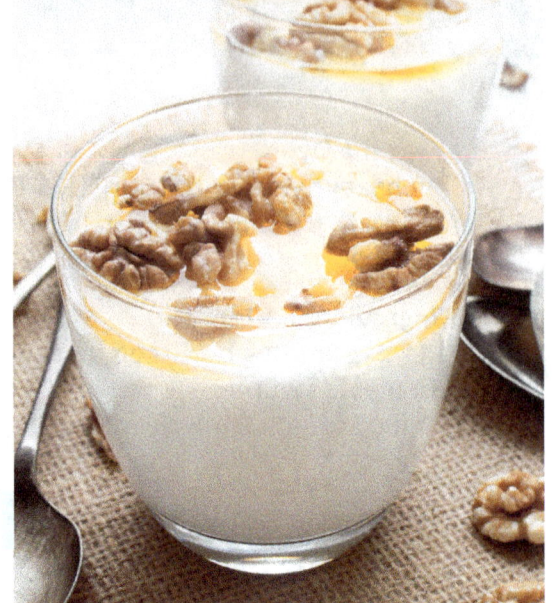

SERVINGS	**2**
Prep Time	**5 min**
Total Time	**5 min**

Calories	Approximately 200 (without added fruit)
Protein	Approximately 8g
Fat	Approximately 10g
Carbohydrates	Approximately 25g
Potassium	Approximately 200mg (varies based on ingredients used)

 ## Ingredients

- 1 cup low-fat plain yogurt (check potassium content; consider low-potassium yogurt alternatives)
- 2 tablespoons honey (or maple syrup, if preferred)
- 1/4 cup low-potassium nuts (such as walnuts, pecans, or sunflower seeds; check potassium content)

Optional
- 1/2 teaspoon cinnamon or vanilla extract for added flavor
- Fresh low-potassium fruit for topping (such as strawberries or blueberries)

ⓘ Instructions

Prepare the Yogurt
- In a medium bowl, add the low-fat plain yogurt.

Add Sweetener
- Drizzle the honey (or maple syrup) over the yogurt. If desired, mix in cinnamon or vanilla extract for additional flavor.

Add Nuts
- Chop the low-potassium nuts if they are whole, and sprinkle them over the yogurt.

Top with Fruit (Optional)
- If using, add a few fresh low-potassium berries on top for extra flavor and nutrition.

Serve
- Serve immediately as a quick breakfast or snack.

Tips

- **Yogurt Options:** Choose a yogurt that is lower in potassium. Greek yogurt can be higher in protein but also higher in potassium, so consider portion size.
- **Nut Selection:** Use nuts that are lower in potassium and adjust the portion based on your dietary needs. If nuts are too high in potassium, consider substituting with seeds like sunflower seeds.
- **Fruit Choices:** When adding fruit, select low-potassium options and use them in moderation to keep potassium levels in check.
- **Storage:** This dish is best enjoyed fresh but can be prepared in advance. Store in an airtight container in the refrigerator for up to 2 days.

MEAL PLANNING FOR SUCCESS

How to Create a Weekly Meal Plan for Low Potassium

Creating a weekly meal plan for a low-potassium diet can help you manage your potassium intake while ensuring that you enjoy a variety of delicious and nutritious meals. Here's a step-by-step guide to help you design an effective meal plan tailored to your dietary needs:

STEP 1
Understand Your Potassium Limits
- *Consult Your Healthcare Provider:* Before starting a low-potassium meal plan, consult with your healthcare provider or registered dietitian to determine your specific potassium intake goals based on your health status and dietary needs.
- *Know High and Low-Potassium Foods:* Familiarize yourself with foods that are high in potassium (e.g., bananas, potatoes, tomatoes) and those that are lower in potassium (e.g., apples, berries, zucchini).

STEP 2
Choose Your Meal Planning Tools
- *Select a Format:* Use a physical planner, a digital app, or a simple spreadsheet to organize your meal plan. Choose a format that works best for you and allows for easy updates.
- *Create a Template:* Design a template for your weekly meal plan that includes sections for breakfast, lunch, dinner, and snacks.

STEP 3
Plan Your Meals

Breakfast Ideas
- Oatmeal with blueberries (made with low-potassium almond milk)
- Egg white omelet with spinach
- Chia seed pudding with low-potassium fruit
- Low-potassium muffins with applesauce

Lunch Ideas
- Quinoa salad with cucumbers and bell peppers
- Grilled chicken salad with lemon dressing
- Vegetable wraps with hummus
- Baked sweet potato with black beans

Dinner Ideas
- Baked cod with herbs and a side of steamed zucchini
- Stir-fried tofu with bell peppers and low-potassium rice
- Grilled salmon with asparagus
- Chicken with lemon and thyme served with roasted root vegetables

Snack Ideas
- Hummus with carrot sticks
- Rice cakes with almond butter
- Low-potassium fruit salad
- Energy bites with oats and honey

STEP 4
Create a Shopping List
- *List Ingredients:* Based on your meal plan, create a shopping list of all the ingredients you will need for the week. Be sure to include low-potassium alternatives.
- *Check Your Pantry:* Before shopping, check your pantry and refrigerator for any items you may already have to avoid duplicate purchases.

STEP 5
Meal Prep
- *Batch Cooking:* Prepare certain ingredients in advance, such as cooking quinoa or rice, chopping vegetables, or making snacks like energy bites or muffins. This will save you time during the week.
- *Storage:* Use airtight containers to store prepped ingredients and meals in the refrigerator for easy access.

Stay Flexible

- *Adjust as Needed:* Be open to adjusting your meal plan based on your schedule, cravings, or availability of ingredients. Flexibility can help you stay committed to your low-potassium diet.
- *Try New Recipes:* Incorporate new recipes or ingredients to keep your meals exciting and enjoyable.

STEP 7
Monitor Your Progress

- *Track Your Potassium Intake:* Keep a journal or use an app to monitor your potassium intake and assess how well you are staying within your limits.
- *Evaluate and Adjust:* At the end of the week, evaluate how well your meal plan worked and make adjustments for the following week as needed.

Creating a weekly meal plan for a low-potassium diet can help you manage your dietary needs while ensuring a variety of tasty meals. By understanding your potassium limits, planning meals, and preparing in advance, you can confidently navigate your dietary restrictions and enjoy nourishing food. Remember to collaborate with healthcare professionals for personalized advice and support as you embark on this journey toward better health.

Tips for Meal Prepping Low Potassium Meals

Meal prepping is an excellent strategy for managing a low-potassium diet, especially for individuals with chronic kidney disease (CKD) or other health conditions that require potassium monitoring. By preparing meals in advance, you can ensure that you have healthy, low-potassium options readily available throughout the week. Here are some effective tips for meal prepping low-potassium meals:

1. Plan Your Meals
- *Create a Weekly Menu:* Start by planning your meals for the week. Include a variety of low-potassium recipes for breakfast, lunch, dinner, and snacks to keep your diet interesting.
- *Utilize a Meal Planning Template:* Use a meal planning template to organize your meals and snacks. This will help you visualize your week and ensure you have everything you need.

2. Choose Low-Potassium Ingredients
- *Know Your Foods:* Familiarize yourself with low-potassium foods and their potassium levels. Focus on incorporating low-potassium fruits, vegetables, grains, and proteins into your meal prep.
- *Make Smart Substitutions:* Opt for lower-potassium alternatives when possible, such as white rice instead of brown rice, or egg whites instead of whole eggs.

3. Batch Cooking
- *Cook in Batches:* Prepare larger quantities of certain foods, such as grains (rice, quinoa), proteins (chicken, turkey, tofu), and vegetables. This allows you to create multiple meals quickly.
- *Use One-Pot Meals:* Consider making one-pot meals or casseroles that can be portioned out for several days. This can save time and reduce the number of dishes to wash.

4. Portion Control

- *Use Portion Containers:* Invest in portion-sized containers to help control serving sizes and make it easier to grab meals on the go. This is especially helpful for maintaining appropriate potassium levels.
- *Label Containers:* Label each container with the meal name and date to keep track of freshness and avoid confusion.

5. Prepare Snacks

- *Healthy Low-Potassium Snacks:* Prepare low-potassium snacks in advance, such as hummus with carrot sticks, rice cakes with almond butter, or low-potassium fruit salad. Portion them into snack-sized containers for easy access.
- *Energy Bites:* Make energy bites ahead of time to have a quick, nutritious snack option ready.

6. Use Freezing Wisely

- *Freeze Meals:* If you prepare large batches, consider freezing individual portions for later use. This is especially useful for soups, stews, and casseroles.
- *Label Freezer Bags:* When freezing meals, use freezer-safe bags or containers and label them with the meal name and date to avoid mix-ups.

7. Utilize Cooking Techniques

- *Incorporate Low-Potassium Cooking Methods:* Use cooking techniques that can help reduce potassium levels, such as boiling or leaching certain vegetables before cooking them.
- *Experiment with Flavor:* Use herbs, spices, and low-sodium flavorings to enhance the taste of your meals without increasing potassium levels.

8. Stay Organized

- *Keep a Meal Prep Schedule:* Set aside specific times each week for meal prepping. Consistency will help establish a routine and make it easier to stay on track.
- *Prepare a Shopping List:* Create a shopping list based on your meal plan to ensure you have all the necessary ingredients on hand.

9. Involve Family Members

- *Get Others Involved:* Involve family members in the meal prep process. This can make cooking more enjoyable and help everyone understand the dietary needs of the individual managing CKD.

10. Evaluate and Adjust

- *Reflect on Your Meal Prep:* At the end of the week, evaluate what worked well and what didn't. Adjust your meal prep strategies based on your experiences to improve the process for the following week.

Meal prepping low-potassium meals can help individuals manage their dietary needs effectively while enjoying a variety of nutritious foods. By planning ahead, choosing the right ingredients, and utilizing efficient cooking methods, you can ensure that you have delicious, kidney-friendly meals ready to enjoy throughout the week. With these tips, you can confidently navigate your low-potassium diet and maintain a healthy lifestyle.

Sample One-Week Low Potassium Meal Plan

This sample one-week low-potassium meal plan is designed to provide balanced nutrition while managing potassium intake. Feel free to adjust portion sizes and ingredients according to your specific dietary needs and preferences.

DAY 1

Breakfast:
- Oatmeal with blueberries (made with low-potassium almond milk)
- 1 tablespoon honey

Lunch:
- Grilled chicken salad with mixed greens, cucumbers, and a lemon dressing
- 1 small apple

Dinner:
- Baked cod with herbs
- Steamed zucchini
- White rice

Snack:
- Hummus with carrot sticks

DAY 2

Breakfast:
- Egg white omelet with spinach and bell peppers
- 1 slice of whole grain toast

Lunch:
- Quinoa salad with diced cucumbers and a drizzle of olive oil
- 1/2 cup low-potassium fruit salad (strawberries, blueberries)

Dinner:
- Stir-fried tofu with bell peppers and broccoli (use low-sodium soy sauce)
- Brown rice (in moderation)

Snack:
- Rice cakes with almond butter

DAY 3

Breakfast:
- Chia seed pudding made with low-potassium almond milk and topped with raspberries

Lunch:
- Vegetable wrap with hummus, spinach, and bell peppers
- 1 small pear

Dinner:
- Chicken with lemon and thyme
- Roasted root vegetables (carrots, turnips)
- Quinoa (in moderation)

Snack:
- Yogurt with honey and chopped walnuts

DAY 4

Breakfast:
- Smoothie with kale, pear, and low-potassium almond milk

Lunch:
- Lentil soup (prepared with low-sodium broth)
- 1 slice of whole grain bread

Dinner:
- Grilled salmon with asparagus
- Mashed cauliflower (instead of potatoes)

Snack:
- Energy bites made with oats and honey

DAY 5

Breakfast:
- Muffins with applesauce (low-potassium recipe)

Lunch:
- Chickpea salad with diced bell peppers and cucumbers
- 1 small apple

Dinner:
- Baked chicken with rosemary
- Steamed green beans
- White rice

Snack:
- Low-potassium fruit salad

DAY 6

Breakfast:
- Overnight oats with almond milk and topped with blueberries

Lunch:
- Quinoa and cucumber salad with lemon vinaigrette
- 1 small orange (in moderation)

Dinner:
- Vegetable curry (with zucchini, bell peppers, and carrots)
- Served with white rice

Snack:
- Yogurt with honey and a sprinkle of cinnamon

DAY 7

Breakfast:
- Savory breakfast muffins (low-potassium recipe)

Lunch:
- Grilled chicken salad with mixed greens, carrots, and low-sodium dressing
- 1/2 cup strawberries

Dinner:
- Beef and broccoli stir-fry with low-sodium soy sauce
- Served over white rice

Snack:
- Coconut macaroons (low-potassium recipe)

Tips for Customizing Your Meal Plan

- Adjust Portions: Depending on your potassium limits, you may need to adjust portion sizes.
- Incorporate Variety: Feel free to swap out ingredients or meals based on availability and personal preferences while keeping potassium in mind.
- Consult with a Dietitian: If you have specific dietary needs or restrictions, consider consulting with a registered dietitian who specializes in renal nutrition for personalized meal planning.

This sample meal plan is intended to help you manage your potassium intake while enjoying a variety of delicious and nutritious meals throughout the week!

COPING WITH DIETARY RESTRICTIONS

Navigating Social Situations with Healthy Meals

Managing a low potassium diet can be challenging, especially in social situations where food is involved. Whether you're attending a family gathering, dining out with friends, or participating in community events, it's essential to feel confident and prepared. Here are some practical tips to help you navigate social situations successfully while adhering to your dietary restrictions:

1. Plan Ahead
- *Know the Venue:* If you're going to a restaurant or event, check the menu online beforehand. Look for low-potassium options, and don't hesitate to call the restaurant to ask about their dishes and how they can accommodate your dietary needs.
- *Bring Your Own Dish:* When invited to a potluck or gathering, consider bringing a low-potassium dish that you can enjoy. This ensures you have at least one safe option and introduces others to delicious kidney-friendly recipes.

2. Communicate Your Needs
- *Inform Hosts or Friends:* Don't hesitate to communicate your dietary restrictions to the host or friends. Most people will appreciate your honesty and may be willing to accommodate your needs by preparing suitable dishes.
- *Ask Questions:* When dining out, ask the server about how dishes are prepared and their ingredients. This can help you make informed choices and avoid high-potassium foods.

3. Make Smart Choices
- *Focus on Low-Potassium Foods:* When presented with food options, prioritize low-potassium foods. Choose items like:
  - Grilled or baked meats (without sauces high in potassium)
  - Low-potassium vegetables (like zucchini, bell peppers, and carrots)
  - White rice or pasta over whole grain options (if potassium is a concern)

- *Portion Control:* If you must eat something higher in potassium, keep the portion small and balance it with low-potassium foods in your meal.

4. Modify Recipes
- *Suggest Alternatives:* If you're cooking for a group or family, suggest modifications to traditional recipes to make them low-potassium. For example, if a dish typically includes potatoes, suggest using mashed cauliflower instead.
- *Share Recipes:* Share some of your favorite low-potassium recipes with friends and family. This can encourage them to try cooking with kidney-friendly ingredients.

5. Stay Mindful at Buffets
- *Survey the Options:* At a buffet, take a moment to survey all the food options before filling your plate. This will help you choose wisely and avoid high-potassium foods.
- *Use Smaller Plates:* If possible, use a smaller plate to help control portion sizes and avoid overwhelming yourself with too many options.

6. Practice Portion Control
- *Be Conscious of Serving Sizes:* Familiarize yourself with appropriate serving sizes for high-potassium foods so you can make informed choices when faced with food options.
- *Balance Your Plate:* Aim to fill your plate with a larger portion of low-potassium foods and smaller portions of higher-potassium foods, if necessary.

7. Stay Flexible and Positive
- *Be Adaptable:* Social situations can be unpredictable. Stay flexible and be prepared to adapt your choices based on what is available.
- *Focus on Enjoyment:* Remember that social gatherings are about more than just food. Focus on enjoying the company of friends and family, engaging in conversations, and celebrating together, rather than solely on the food.

8. Carry Snacks

- *Pack Healthy Snacks:* If you're going to an event where food options may be limited, consider bringing low-potassium snacks with you. This ensures you have something safe to eat if suitable options aren't available.
- *Stay Nourished:* Having snacks on hand can help you avoid hunger and make it easier to resist high-potassium foods.

Navigating social situations with a low potassium diet may require some planning and communication, but it is entirely manageable. By being proactive, making informed choices, and focusing on the social aspects of gatherings, you can enjoy your time with friends and family while staying true to your dietary needs. Remember, you are not alone in this journey; support from loved ones and healthcare professionals can make a significant difference in successfully managing your low potassium diet.

Involving Family in Meal Preparation

Involving family members in meal preparation can be a fun and rewarding experience, especially for individuals managing a low-potassium diet due to chronic kidney disease (CKD) or other health conditions. Engaging loved ones not only fosters a supportive environment but also helps educate them about dietary needs and encourages healthy eating habits for the entire household. Here are several effective strategies for involving family in meal preparation:

1. Educate and Inform

- *Share Your Dietary Needs:* Begin by explaining your dietary restrictions and the importance of managing potassium levels. This will help your family understand the significance of the meal preparation process and encourage their support.
- *Discuss Low-Potassium Foods:* Introduce family members to low-potassium foods and explain which items should be limited or avoided. This knowledge will empower them to make informed choices while cooking.

2. Plan Meals Together

- *Collaborative Meal Planning:* Sit down with your family to create a weekly meal plan. Encourage everyone to contribute their favorite low-potassium recipes and ideas, helping to foster a sense of involvement and ownership.
- *Explore New Recipes:* Use this opportunity to explore new low-potassium recipes together. This can make meal planning more exciting and introduce your family to a variety of healthy options.

3. Assign Roles in Meal Prep

- *Divide Responsibilities:* Assign specific tasks to family members based on their interests and skills. For example, one person can handle chopping vegetables, while another can prepare the protein or cook the grains.

- *Involve Kids in Cooking:* Encourage children to participate in meal preparation by assigning age-appropriate tasks, such as washing vegetables, stirring mixtures, or setting the table. This involvement helps instill healthy cooking habits from a young age.

4. Make Cooking a Family Activity
- *Cook Together:* Set aside time for family cooking sessions where everyone can gather in the kitchen. Cooking together can be a fun bonding experience and allows for creativity in the kitchen.
- *Create a Cooking Playlist:* Play music while you cook to make the experience enjoyable and lively. This can help create a positive atmosphere and make meal prep feel less like a chore.

5. Teach Cooking Techniques
- *Share Cooking Skills:* Use this opportunity to teach family members cooking techniques that are particularly beneficial for low-potassium meal preparation, such as leaching and boiling vegetables to reduce potassium content.
- *Encourage Experimentation:* Allow family members to experiment with different spices, herbs, and cooking methods to enhance the flavor of low-potassium dishes. This encourages creativity and helps everyone feel invested in the cooking process.

6. Prepare Snacks Together
- *Healthy Snack Prep:* Involve family in preparing healthy low-potassium snacks, such as energy bites, yogurt parfaits, or vegetable sticks with hummus. Having nutritious snacks on hand can support everyone's health and make it easier to stick to dietary goals.

7. Establish a Routine
- *Regular Meal Prep Sessions:* Create a regular schedule for meal prep, such as Sundays for the upcoming week. This routine can help keep everyone engaged and make it easier to plan and prepare meals.
- *Rotate Responsibilities:* Allow different family members to take turns leading meal prep sessions or planning meals. This rotation keeps everyone involved and allows for sharing of cooking styles and preferences.

8. Celebrate Your Efforts

- *Enjoy Family Meals:* After preparing meals together, make it a point to sit down and enjoy family meals. This reinforces the importance of shared meals and the effort everyone has put into preparing them.
- *Acknowledge Contributions:* Recognize and appreciate each family member's contributions in the kitchen. Positive reinforcement encourages continued participation and fosters a supportive cooking environment.

Involving family in meal preparation is a valuable strategy for managing a low-potassium diet. By educating loved ones, planning meals together, and sharing responsibilities, you create a supportive environment that fosters healthy eating habits for everyone. Cooking can become a fun and engaging family activity, making it easier to navigate dietary restrictions while enjoying delicious, nutritious meals together. Embrace the opportunity to bond with your family through cooking and celebrate the shared commitment to health and well-being.

Cooking for Mixed Dietary Needs

Cooking for a family or group with mixed dietary needs can be a rewarding yet challenging task, especially when managing restrictions such as a low-potassium diet alongside other dietary preferences or restrictions (like vegetarianism, gluten-free, or allergies). Here are some practical strategies to help you successfully navigate cooking for diverse dietary needs while ensuring everyone enjoys delicious meals.

1. Understand Everyone's Needs
- *Gather Information:* Start by discussing dietary restrictions, preferences, and allergies with everyone involved. Understanding what each person can and cannot eat is essential for successful meal planning.
- *Identify Common Goals:* While different dietary needs may exist, look for commonalities. For example, many diets emphasize whole foods, vegetables, and lean proteins, which can serve as a foundation for meal planning.

2. Plan Inclusive Meals
- *Choose Versatile Dishes:* Opt for recipes that can be easily adapted to meet different dietary needs. For example, stir-fries, salads, or grain bowls can be customized with various proteins and vegetables.
- *Create Build-Your-Own Meals:* Consider meals where everyone can assemble their own plates, such as tacos, wraps, or grain bowls. Provide a variety of low-potassium and other options, allowing individuals to choose what suits their dietary needs.

3. Prepare Ingredients Separately
- *Cook Components Individually:* When preparing mixed-diet meals, consider cooking certain components separately. For example, cook low-potassium grains or proteins separately from higher-potassium options, allowing family members to combine them according to their preferences.

- *Use Separate Cooking Utensils:* To avoid cross-contamination, use separate cutting boards, utensils, and cooking pots for different dietary needs, particularly for allergens or strict dietary restrictions.

4. Focus on Low-Potassium Ingredients

- *Use Low-Potassium Alternatives:* When planning meals, prioritize low-potassium ingredients that can be enjoyed by everyone. For example, use low-potassium vegetables (like zucchini, bell peppers, and carrots) in dishes that can accommodate various diets.
- *Healthy Substitutions:* Explore alternatives for high-potassium ingredients. For example, use white rice instead of brown rice, or substitute high-potassium fruits with lower-potassium options.

5. Incorporate Flavorful Herbs and Spices

- *Enhance Flavor Without Salt:* Use herbs, spices, and citrus to add flavor to dishes without relying on high-sodium or high-potassium ingredients. This approach can enhance the overall taste of meals, making them enjoyable for everyone.

6. Label and Organize

- *Label Dishes Clearly:* If you prepare multiple dishes, label them according to dietary needs (e.g., "low potassium," "vegetarian," "gluten-free"). This helps family members easily identify what they can eat.
- *Organize the Buffet Style:* If serving a variety of options, consider a buffet-style setup where everyone can choose their preferred dishes. This allows for personalization and accommodates diverse dietary preferences.

7. Plan Ahead for Special Occasions

- *Discuss Menu Options:* For family gatherings or special occasions, discuss the menu well in advance. This allows everyone to contribute ideas and ensures that all dietary needs are considered.
- *Prepare a Variety of Dishes:* When hosting a meal, aim to prepare a range of dishes that cater to various dietary needs. Ensure there are enough low-potassium options to satisfy those on restricted diets while also providing choices for others.

8. Encourage Family Participation

- *Involve Everyone in Cooking:* Encourage family members to participate in meal preparation. This can be a fun way to teach everyone about different dietary needs and promote understanding and cooperation.
- *Cook Together:* Make cooking a family activity, allowing everyone to contribute to the meal. This not only fosters teamwork but also creates opportunities for learning and experimentation in the kitchen.

Cooking for mixed dietary needs requires careful planning, creativity, and open communication. By understanding everyone's dietary restrictions, planning inclusive meals, and preparing adaptable dishes, you can create a harmonious cooking environment that satisfies the diverse preferences of family and friends. Embrace the opportunity to learn from each other and celebrate the joy of sharing meals together, ensuring that everyone feels included and nourished.

ADDITIONAL RESOURCES

Recommended Kidney Health and Nutrition Websites

For individuals managing chronic kidney disease (CKD) or those interested in kidney health and nutrition, reliable information is crucial. The following websites offer valuable resources, educational materials, and support for patients, caregivers, and healthcare providers alike.

1. **National Kidney Foundation (NKF)**
- Website: *www.kidney.org*
- Overview: The NKF provides comprehensive information on kidney health, including resources on chronic kidney disease, dietary guidelines, and patient education materials. They also offer tools like the Kidney Disease Outcomes Quality Initiative (KDOQI) guidelines.

2. **American Association of Kidney Patients (AAKP)**
- Website: *www.aakp.org*
- Overview: AAKP is dedicated to improving the quality of life for kidney patients. Their website offers educational resources, advocacy information, and a community forum for patients and caregivers to connect.

3. **Kidney Disease: Improving Global Outcomes (KDIGO)**
- Website: *www.kdigo.org*
- Overview: KDIGO provides clinical practice guidelines for managing kidney diseases globally. Their resources are geared toward healthcare professionals but are also useful for patients seeking evidence-based information.

4. American Kidney Fund (AKF)
- Website: *www.kidneyfund.org*
- Overview: The AKF provides information on kidney disease prevention, treatment options, and financial assistance for those affected by kidney disease. They also have a section dedicated to nutrition and meal planning.

5. National Institute of Diabetes and Digestive and Kidney Diseases (NIDDK)
- Website: *www.niddk.nih.gov*
- Overview: NIDDK offers a wealth of information on kidney diseases, including research findings, educational materials, and dietary guidelines tailored for kidney health.

6. The Kidney Community Kitchen
- Website: *www.kidneycommunitykitchen.ca*
- Overview: This site provides kidney-friendly recipes and nutrition information specifically designed for people living with kidney disease. It offers practical tips for meal preparation and planning.

7. RenalTracker
- Website: *https://blog.renaltracker.com/*
- Overview: Clear, evidence-based, and personally relevant information on giving CKD a place in your life – without all the conflicting info you may find online.

These websites serve as valuable resources for individuals seeking information on kidney health and nutrition. Whether you are a patient, caregiver, or healthcare professional, these organizations provide evidence-based guidelines, recipes, and support to help you navigate the challenges of managing kidney disease effectively.

Support Groups and Community Resources

Navigating the challenges of chronic kidney disease (CKD) can be overwhelming, but you don't have to face it alone. Support groups and community resources provide essential emotional, educational, and practical support for individuals living with CKD and their families. Here are some valuable resources to consider:

1. **American Association of Kidney Patients (AAKP)**
- Website: *www.aakp.org*
- Overview: AAKP offers various support resources, including online forums, educational materials, and advocacy programs. They provide information on local support groups and host events that bring patients and caregivers together.

2. **National Kidney Foundation (NKF)**
- Website: *www.kidney.org*
- Overview: The NKF has a network of local chapters that offer support groups, educational programs, and community events. Their resources include educational materials tailored for patients and families.

3. **Kidney Community Kitchen**
- Website: *www.kidneycommunitykitchen.ca*
- Overview: This resource offers not only recipes but also community support and workshops focused on kidney health and nutrition. It connects individuals with others who share similar dietary challenges.

4. Renal Support Network (RSN)

- Website: *www.rsnhope.org*
- Overview: RSN provides peer support through various programs, including online support groups, educational webinars, and community events. Their focus is on empowering patients to take charge of their health.

5. Kidney Disease: Improving Global Outcomes (KDIGO)

- Website: *www.kdigo.org*
- Overview: KDIGO provides guidelines and resources for healthcare professionals and patients. While primarily focused on clinical practice, they also offer educational material that can be helpful for individuals seeking to understand their condition.

9. National Kidney Foundation's Kidney Walks

- Website: *www.kidney.org/kidneywalk*
- Overview: The NKF organizes Kidney Walks across the country to raise awareness and funds for kidney health. Participating in these events can connect you with others in the kidney community and provide support.

Support groups and community resources are vital for individuals managing chronic kidney disease. They provide essential emotional support, education, and practical advice, helping patients and their families feel less isolated in their journey. By connecting with others who understand the challenges of CKD, you can gain valuable insights, share experiences, and foster a sense of community. Remember, you are not alone—support is available to help you navigate your health journey effectively.

CONCLUSION

Empowering Your Journey to Manage Potassium Levels

Managing potassium levels is a vital aspect of living with chronic kidney disease (CKD) or other related conditions. While dietary restrictions may seem daunting, understanding the importance of potassium management and implementing effective strategies can empower you on your health journey. Here are key points to help you navigate this process confidently:

1. Understanding Potassium's Role

- *Essential Mineral:* Potassium is crucial for various bodily functions, including muscle contractions, nerve signaling, and fluid balance. However, when kidney function declines, the body may struggle to excrete excess potassium, making management essential.
- *Know Your Limits:* Consult your healthcare provider or registered dietitian to determine your specific potassium intake goals based on your health status. Understanding your limits is the first step in effectively managing your diet.

2. Educate Yourself

- *Learn About Potassium:* Familiarize yourself with high-potassium foods (e.g., bananas, potatoes, tomatoes) and low-potassium alternatives (e.g., apples, berries, zucchini). This knowledge will empower you to make informed dietary choices.
- *Read Labels:* Get into the habit of checking food labels for potassium content. Many processed foods can contain hidden sources of potassium, so being vigilant is crucial.

3. Plan Your Meals

- *Create a Weekly Meal Plan:* Planning meals in advance can help you stay organized and ensure you're incorporating a variety of low-potassium foods. Use resources like cookbooks and online recipes to find kidney-friendly options.
- *Batch Cooking:* Prepare larger quantities of low-potassium meals and snacks. This not only saves time but also ensures you have nutritious options readily available.

4. Incorporate Cooking Techniques

- *Use Cooking Methods to Reduce Potassium:* Techniques like leaching (soaking) and boiling can help reduce the potassium content of certain foods. Familiarize yourself with these methods to make the most of your ingredients.
- *Experiment with Flavor:* Use herbs, spices, and citrus to enhance the flavor of low-potassium dishes. This will help you enjoy your meals without feeling deprived.

5. Monitor Your Progress

- *Regular Testing:* Schedule regular blood tests to monitor your potassium levels and assess the effectiveness of your dietary changes. This will help you and your healthcare team make necessary adjustments.
- *Keep a Food Diary:* Consider maintaining a food diary to track your potassium intake and identify patterns in your eating habits. This can provide valuable insights into your dietary choices.

6. Seek Support

- *Engage with Healthcare Professionals:* Working with healthcare providers, including nephrologists and registered dietitians, can provide tailored guidance and support. Don't hesitate to reach out for help when needed.
- *Join Support Groups:* Connecting with others who are managing similar dietary restrictions can provide emotional support and practical tips. Consider joining local or online support groups focused on kidney health.

7. Involve Your Family

- *Educate Family Members:* Share your dietary needs with family and friends. Educating them about potassium management can help foster a supportive environment where everyone understands your dietary choices.
- *Cook Together:* Involve family members in meal preparation. Cooking together can create a sense of teamwork and help everyone learn about low-potassium options.

8. Stay Positive and Flexible

- *Embrace the Journey:* Managing potassium levels is an ongoing process. Approach it with a positive mindset and be open to learning and adapting as you go.
- *Celebrate Small Wins:* Acknowledge your progress, whether it's trying a new recipe or successfully navigating a social situation. Celebrating these small victories can keep you motivated.

Empowering yourself to manage potassium levels effectively involves education, planning, and support. By understanding the role of potassium, making informed dietary choices, and utilizing practical strategies, you can take control of your health and enjoy a fulfilling life. Remember, you are not alone on this journey—seek support, stay informed, and embrace the opportunities to learn and grow as you navigate your dietary needs. With the right knowledge and resources, you can thrive while managing your potassium intake!

Thank You and Encouragement for Healthy Living

As you embark on your journey to manage potassium levels and improve your overall health, we want to take a moment to express our gratitude and provide you with encouragement. Your commitment to making dietary changes and prioritizing your health is commendable, and it's important to recognize the strength and resilience you possess.

Thank You for Your Commitment

Thank you for choosing to invest in your health by exploring The Essential Low Potassium Cookbook. By seeking out information and resources, you are taking proactive steps toward managing your condition and enhancing your quality of life. It's not always easy to navigate dietary restrictions, but your dedication to learning and adapting is a powerful testament to your determination.

Embrace the Journey

Remember that managing a low-potassium diet is a journey, not a destination. There will be challenges along the way, but each step you take brings you closer to achieving your health goals. Embrace this journey with an open mind and a positive attitude. Celebrate your successes, no matter how small, and learn from any setbacks you encounter.

Focus on Enjoyment

- Eating should be an enjoyable experience, and it's possible to savor delicious meals while adhering to your dietary restrictions. Explore new recipes, experiment with flavors, and involve your family in the cooking process. By making meal preparation a fun and engaging activity, you can transform the way you think about food and health.

Build a Support Network
Surround yourself with a supportive community. Whether it's family, friends, or fellow individuals managing CKD, having a network of people who understand your journey can make a significant difference. Share your experiences, seek advice, and encourage one another in making healthy choices.

Stay Informed and Adaptable
Continue to educate yourself about kidney health and nutrition. Stay informed about the latest research, dietary guidelines, and cooking techniques that can enhance your meals. Be adaptable in your approach; as you learn more about your dietary needs, you may discover new foods and recipes that fit well within your potassium limits.

Prioritize Self-Care
In addition to managing your diet, prioritize self-care and overall well-being. Engage in activities that bring you joy, practice stress management techniques, and ensure you are taking care of your mental and emotional health. Your well-being is a holistic journey that encompasses both physical and mental health.

As you move forward on this path, remember that you have the power to take control of your health. By making informed dietary choices and embracing a low-potassium lifestyle, you are investing in your future well-being. Thank you for allowing The Essential Low Potassium Cookbook to be a part of your journey, and we wish you success as you continue to explore and enjoy the many flavors of healthy living.
Stay hopeful, stay inspired, and most importantly, enjoy the journey toward a healthier you!

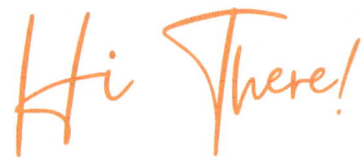

Hi There!

I hope you are enjoying my book so far. I would really appreciate it if you could leave a quick review on Amazon.

Just simply scan the code below using your mobile phone's camera, or you can enter the link below on our web browser.

https://go.renaltracker.com/LowPotassiumCookbook

Thanks a lot!

-Janeth

INDEX